Legal and Ethical Issues for Health Professions

Legal and Ethical Issues for Health Professions

THIRD EDITION

Jeanne McTeigue, CPC, CPC-I
Medical Billing and Coding Chairperson
Branford Hall Career Institute
Albany, New York

Christopher Lee, CST, FAST
Surgical Technologist
Northwestern Memorial Hospital
Chicago, Illinois

KH

SAUNDERS

3251 Riverport Lane
St. Louis, Missouri 63043

LEGAL AND ETHICAL ISSUES FOR HEALTH PROFESSIONS,
THIRD EDITION

ISBN: 978-1-4557-3366-8

Notices

Knowledge and best practice in this field are constantly changing. As new research and experience broaden our understanding, changes in research methods, professional practices, or medical treatment may become necessary.

Practitioners and researchers must always rely on their own experience and knowledge in evaluating and using any information, methods, compounds, or experiments described herein. In using such information or methods they should be mindful of their own safety and the safety of others, including parties for whom they have a professional responsibility.

With respect to any drug or pharmaceutical products identified, readers are advised to check the most current information provided (i) on procedures featured or (ii) by the manufacturer of each product to be administered, to verify the recommended dose or formula, the method and duration of administration, and contraindications. It is the responsibility of practitioners, relying on their own experience and knowledge of their patients, to make diagnoses, to determine dosages and the best treatment for each individual patient, and to take all appropriate safety precautions.

To the fullest extent of the law, neither the Publisher nor the authors, contributors, or editors, assume any liability for any injury and/or damage to persons or property as a matter of products liability, negligence or otherwise, or from any use or operation of any methods, products, instructions, or ideas contained in the material herein.

ISBN: 978-1-4557-3366-8

Executive Content Strategist: Jennifer Janson
Senior Content Development Specialist: Jennifer Bertucci
Publishing Services Manager: Jeffrey Patterson
Senior Project Manager: Jeanne Genz
Designer: Amy Buxton

Printed in the United States of America

Last digit is the print number: 9 8 7 6 5 4 3 2

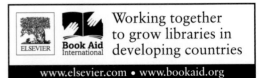

2/23/16

Reviewers

Virginia M. Mishkin, MS, RT(R)(M)(QM)
Program Director, Radiologic Technology Program
Bronx Community College of The City University of New York
Bronx, New York

Jennifer Reisinger, MHRM
Lead Instructor
Miami-Jacobs Career College
Dayton, Ohio

Jeanne Sewell, MSN, RN-BC
Assistant Professor, School of Nursing
Georgia College & State University
Milledgeville, Georgia

Preface

The purpose of the third edition of *Legal and Ethical Issues for Health Professions* is to provide health professionals with a comprehensive, user-friendly textbook and reference that focuses on the legal and ethical issues faced by them on a day-to-day, real-life basis. The writing style is approachable, the case studies are plentiful, and the information is wide-ranging and applicable.

Many changes have been implemented to this third edition—the design and format are now full-color, making the book much more visually appealing. Also, the chapters have been reorganized into an even more logical format; Chapter 1 discusses the U.S. Legal System, and then we move on to The Basics of Ethics, which rounds out the introductory material. From there, various types of legal and ethical issues as well as common areas of liability and litigation are discussed in a rational, consistent manner. For this edition, separate chapters are provided for the following: ethical and bioethical issues, workplace issues, code and standards infractions, the medical malpractice lawsuit and the trial process, intentional and quasi-intentional torts, statutory reporting and public duties, professional liability insurance, death and dying issues, conflict management, and business aspects of healthcare. Chapters have been restructured, rewritten, reorganized, and repurposed, and this third edition brings together all the applicable legal and ethical issues in the current world of health professions.

Features

With this new edition brings many helpful new features with up-to-date information, applicable questions that require critical thinking, and real-life, relatable scenarios. Some of these valuable learning aids include the following:

- **Key Terms** are identified and defined at the beginning of each chapter, providing students with a valuable terminology overview for each chapter.

KEY TERMS

Administrative law Codifies interactions between citizens and government agencies, provides certain police power to the agencies to enforce the regulations, and governs the agencies themselves.

Admissions of fact Discovery technique that asks the opposing party (in writing) to admit or deny any material fact or the authenticity of documents to be introduced into evidence at trial.

Appellate court A court that hears appeals from lower court decisions; sometimes called court of appeals.

- **Chapter Objectives** are listed at the beginning of each chapter, giving both students and instructors definitive evaluation tools to use as each chapter's content is covered.

CHAPTER OBJECTIVES

1. Define law.
2. Identify specific sources of law.
3. Describe the differences among the U.S. executive, judiciary, and legislative branches.
4. Explain different types of law in the United States.
5. Explain key U.S. laws affecting healthcare professionals.
6. Demonstrate understanding of the various levels of the U.S. court system.

- **Discussion boxes** provide topical discussion questions that will generate beneficial classroom dialogue and compel students to think about topics a bit deeper in order to relate to the real world of health professions.

Discussion
Patient A is seen for a similar diagnosis as patient B, but patient A has a different insurance plan than patient B. Should patient A be treated differently than patient B? Is it a legal issue or an ethical issue if they are treated differently?

- **Relate to Practice scenarios** are designed to assist the student in responding to realistic situations that occur in the life of a health professional.

Relate to Practice
An EMT is loyal to his company because of his own virtues and set of values. The employer treats this EMT unfairly by not bothering to reward this employee with raises, increased benefits, fairness in assigning days off, or other recognition, or worse by mistreating that employee. Who bears responsibility? Who is wrong: the employer for unfair manipulation or the employee for loyalty?

- **What If? questions** present students with real-life ethical dilemmas that they may encounter in the workplace.

What If?
You witness a coworker openly treating a patient disrespectfully because of his or her personal opinion of the patient. If the patient feels that he or she is being treated in a disrespectful or discriminating fashion, the patient could very well make a complaint or claim against the provider. What would you do if you witnessed this happening?

- **Self-Reflection Questions** are placed at the end of every chapter to provide students with pertinent questions that can be used to analyze and evaluate various legal and ethical issues.

Self-Reflection Questions
1. Discuss the reasons and goals of the law.
2. Discuss how the law changes.
3. Discuss how the various sources of law might interact or affect one another.
4. Describe the differences between civil, criminal, and administrative law.

- **Internet Activities** are positioned at the end of every chapter to give students additional topics to research and investigate.

Internet Activities

1. Go to the law library or use the Internet to obtain a copy of an actual case in your area of practice. (Use recommended websites.)
2. Investigate the medical practice acts for your state online and review procedures for licensing.

- **Additional Resources** are listed at the end of some chapters to offer students a chance to take their learning a step further.

Additional Resources

www.findlaw.com
www.lexisone.com or www.lexisnexis.com/community/portal/ (To research cases a
    fee is charged. Other information from the site is still free.)
www.usa.gov
www.definitions.uslegal.com

- **Chapter Review Questions** accompany every chapter and greatly enhance the learning value of the textbook by providing appropriate topic-specific questions so that students can test their retention of each chapter's content.

Chapter Review Questions

1. One of the four elements of negligence is
   A. dereliction of duty.
   B. deliberate act.
   C. Defendant.
   D. executive branch.

Appendixes

This third edition also provides five different helpful appendices to allow for maximum utilization in the classroom of health professionals. Appendix A is a Resource Section that lists many national and state boards that are applicable to modern-day health professionals. Appendix B lists out the general 7-step process of a trial. Appendix C lists 14 different actual case examples that can be used as discussion items, or as supplemental legal coverage. Appendix D includes 14 different case studies that have accompanying questions, which can be used within a course or as additional practice. Appendix E contains 17 supplemental fictional case scenarios that also have accompanying, thought-provoking, situational-type questions for students.

Evolve Resources

The Evolve site (http://evolve.elsevier.com/healthprofessions/legalissues/) includes all instructor materials (TEACH Lesson Plans, TEACH PowerPoint slides, TEACH Answer Keys, and Test Banks, which are for instructors only) as well as sample legal documents, all five appendixes from this textbook, and electronic flashcards of each chapter's key terms, which can be used as study tools.

Acknowledgments

I would like to thank my husband Danny Gandara for guiding, listening to, putting up with, begging, bribing, pleading, threatening, cajoling, and most importantly believing in me. Your support means everything to me and I would not have been able to finish this work without it. I love you!

I would also like to thank Sherri Alexander for seeing something in me that I did not see myself and getting me started on this project. Your friendship has been one of the greatest gifts I have ever received and I will always treasure it.

And I cannot forget the team at Elsevier. Kelly Glogovac, Jennifer Janson, and Jennifer Bertucci, I appreciate all of your hard work and patience with the thousands of questions I asked. Your knowledge and professionalism made this first-time writing experience a pleasant one and I thank you for everything you did for me.

Christopher Lee, CST, FAST

First and foremost I would like to thank the team at Elsevier for this awesome opportunity. Thanks to Kelly Glogovac, Jennifer Janson, and especially Jennifer Bertucci for all your guidance and expertise and for believing in me. An extra special thanks to the best editor, Linda Wendling, that any author (especially a first-timer) could ask for. Thanks for all your patience and mentorship through this project.

I also want to thank my family and especially my children for all the love and support that they always give me and thank them for always encouraging me to be the best I can be, and a special dedication to my grandchildren—all my love to each of you.

This has been a wonderful experience, and as an instructor in this topic I truly hope that all students and instructors using this text will enjoy it as much as we have had creating it.

Jeanne McTeigue, CPC, CPC-I

The publisher would also like to thank Tonia Dandry Aiken for her contributions to this edition—the sample legal documents on the Evolve site, as well as the sample case studies, case discussions, and case scenarios used in the appendixes.

Contents

Chapter 1

The U.S. Legal System

Jeanne McTeigue

KEY TERMS

Administrative law Codifies interactions between citizens and government agencies, provides certain police power to the agencies to enforce the regulations, and governs the agencies themselves.

Admissions of fact Discovery technique that asks the opposing party (in writing) to admit or deny any material fact or the authenticity of documents to be introduced into evidence at trial.

Appellate court A court that hears appeals from lower court decisions; sometimes called court of appeals.

Assault A threat or attempt to inflict offensive physical contact or bodily harm on a person that puts the person in immediate danger of or in apprehension of such harm or contact.

Battery Bodily harm or unlawful touching of another. In the medical field, treating the patient without consent is considered battery.

Civil code Comprehensive collection of private laws, usually including common private laws such as those concerning contracts, torts, property, inheritance, and family issues; as opposed to corporate law.

Civil lawsuit A noncriminal lawsuit for damages, usually based in tort, contract, labor, or privacy.

Common law Law of precedents built on a case-by-case basis and established by citing interpretation of existing laws by judges in previous suits. Also known as "judge made law."

Criminal law State or federal government law covering violations of written criminal code or statute.

Defendant Person or entity sued.

Discovery Process of gathering information in preparation for trial.

Executive branch President of the United States or Governor of an individual state. Can propose laws, veto laws proposed by the legislature, enforce laws, and establish agencies.

Federal court Court having jurisdiction over cases in which the U.S. Constitution and federal statutes apply; these can be federal district courts (trial courts), district courts of appeals, or the U.S. Supreme Court.

Felony Serious crime punishable by relatively large fines and/or imprisonment for more than 1 year and, in some cases, death.

In personam **jurisdiction** A court's power to adjudicate cases filed against a specific individual, as opposed to *in rem* jurisdiction, which concerns property disputes.

In rem **jurisdiction** A term that delineates the court's jurisdiction over property or things, including marriage, rather than over persons.

Interrogatory Pretrial set of written questions that must be answered in writing under oath and returned within a given time frame.

Judicial branch Federal constitutional court system; one of the three parts of the U.S. Federal Government; interprets legislation and determines its constitutionality and applies it to specific cases. May overrule cases presented on appeal from lower courts.

Jurisdiction Authority given by law to a court to try cases and rule on legal matters within a particular geographic area and/or over certain types of legal cases.

Law The foundation of statutes, rules, and regulations that governs people, relationships, behaviors, and interactions with the state, society, and federal government.

Legislative branch The U.S. House of Representatives and Senate and any similar state legislature that develops statutory law.

Malpractice The failure of a professional to meet the standard of conduct that a reasonable and prudent member of the profession would exercise in similar circumstances; it results in harm.

Medical ethics Principles based on the medical profession that determine moral behavior.

Medical law Laws that are prescribed specifically pertaining to the medical field.

Medicare fraud Providing false information to claim medical reimbursements beyond the scope of payment for actual healthcare services rendered.

Misdemeanor Lesser crime punishable by usually modest fines or penalties established by the state or federal government and/or imprisonment of less than 1 year.

Negligence The failure to use such care as a reasonably prudent and careful person would use under similar circumstances; an act of omission or failure to do what a person of ordinary prudence would have done under similar circumstances.

Plaintiff The person or entity bringing a suit or claim.

Request for production of documents A discovery tool whereby requests are submitted to the opposing party to produce specific documents or items that are pertinent to the issues of the case.

Res ipsa loquitur In Latin: "the thing speaks for itself." Legal indication that there is clear proof that the defendant had the responsibility (duty) to the patient and that the injury would not and could not have occurred without the negligence of the defendant.

Standard of care The average knowledge and expertise that one can expect from a healthcare professional in the same area or field and with the same base of training.

Stare decisis In Latin: "to stand by the things decided" or to adhere to a decided case; condition in which, once a court rules, that decision becomes law for other cases. Also known as *precedent*.

State supreme court Highest court in any given state in the U.S. court system.

Statute of limitations Defense against a tort action; requires that a claim be filed within a specific amount of time of discovering that a wrong has been committed.

Tort A wrongful act, not including a breach of contract or trust, that results in injury to another's person, property, reputation, or the like, and for which the injured party is entitled to compensation.

United States Supreme Court Highest court in the United States, having ultimate judicial authority within the United States to interpret and decide questions of federal law. It is head of the judicial branch of the United States Government.

Writ of certiorari Order a higher court issues to review the decision and proceedings in a lower court and determine whether there were any irregularities.

CHAPTER OBJECTIVES

1. Define law.
2. Identify specific sources of law.
3. Describe the differences among the U.S. executive, judiciary, and legislative branches.
4. Explain different types of law in the United States.
5. Explain key U.S. laws affecting healthcare professionals.
6. Demonstrate understanding of the various levels of the U.S. court system.

Introduction

Allied healthcare professionals face a wide range of legal responsibilities to their patients and society, and are bound by laws and regulations the general population does not routinely encounter. Having an understanding about the sources of laws, the types of law, the differences between civil and criminal laws, and the elements of neglect helps to ensure allied healthcare professionals make sound decisions concerning their role in providing quality patient care. A further investigation into the court systems also provides a better understanding of how the law is enforced in general and specific situations, and where the jurisdiction to enforce the law resides.

Every job, profession, and career has a distinct vocabulary. Once you are familiar with the vocabulary, ideas, and concepts, the structure of the job becomes understandable. This chapter reviews the major legal concepts and terms that will aid in the understanding of how legal responsibility affects a healthcare provider.

What Is the Law?

The term law refers to any collection of statutes, rules, and regulations that govern people, relationships, behaviors, and interactions with a state, society, or nation; there are even recognized *international laws* agreed on by a group of nations through treaties and resolutions. Law is meant to provide order in negotiating conflicts among individuals, corporations, states, and other entities. The goal of law is to resolve disputes without violence and to protect the health, safety, and welfare of individual citizens.

In the United States, as in other nations, law—although based on solid, long-held tenets, customs, and beliefs—is constantly evolving and growing to meet the changes, challenges, and constant shifts of our society. For example, the past century has seen different groups in society empowered by laws changed to meet the ever-evolving social, political, technological, and personal values of society (e.g., laws covering the validity of same-sex marriages or the right to drive while texting). By contrast, however, the law is generally more consistent about the caring for others in a healthcare setting. These laws are far less ambiguous and reflect the "ethics" of the society in which they apply. Medical ethics is the judgment that healthcare providers use to determine whether an action should be allowed on the basis of "right and wrong"; therefore, not all unethical acts are always illegal acts. Medical law, however, dictates both the responsibilities of the healthcare provider and the rights of the patient.

> **Discussion**
> Patient A is seen for a similar diagnosis as patient B, but patient A has a different insurance plan than patient B. Should patient A be treated differently than patient B? Is it a legal issue or an ethical issue if they are treated differently?

Sources of Law

In the United States, laws originate from a variety of sources. The primary sources include specific government bodies, important historical documents that are the foundation of our nation, and also specific processes and actions that occur within the court systems.

Branches of Government

The three branches of government provide the basic sources of law (Box 1-1). They are the legislative, executive, and judicial branches. The first branch—the legislature—consists of the House of Representatives and the Senate of the United States and any similar state legislature (Figure 1-1). This branch develops statutory law. These laws are codified and impact all citizens of that state. The Medicare and Medicaid amendments to the Social Security Act of 1965 have dramatically affected healthcare, particularly in the variety of services available in hospitals, communities, and the home; in the number of hospital admissions and discharges; and in the level of care provided.

The second branch of government is the executive branch. The President or Governor proposes legislative action to be taken by individual legislators, either vetoes or approves laws agreed upon by the legislature, and enforces the laws. The executive branch also proposes and establishes certain agencies to enact rules and regulations that become administrative law. Once the legislature creates a statute, it empowers

---

BOX 1-1
Four Sources of Law

Constitution and Bill of Rights
Common law or case law—Judicial branch
Statutory law—Legislative branch
Administrative law—Executive branch

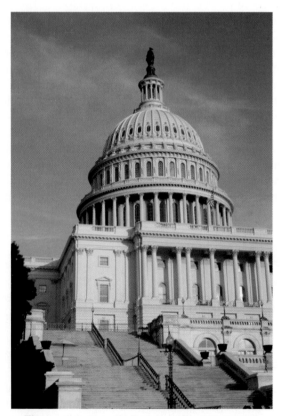

Figure 1-1 Steps leading up to the U.S. Capitol.

the appropriate executive agency to implement and establish rules and regulations to meet the intent of the statute. These rules and regulations codify the interactions between the citizens and the agencies, provide for certain police powers to the agencies to enforce the regulations, and govern the agencies themselves. For example, the rules and regulations of the Occupational Safety and Health Administration (OSHA) apply to most workplaces, including healthcare facilities. Another agency that regulates healthcare workplaces is the U.S. Department of Public Health (DPH), which surveys nursing homes, hospitals, and other healthcare facilities to establish regulations and to enforce compliance with those regulations. The Nurse Practice Acts of the various states create administrative agencies, such as the state boards of nursing, which have the authority to make and enforce rules and regulations concerning nursing practice. Likewise, the boards of medical examiners enforce rules and regulations that affect medical practice.

Finally, the third branch is the judicial system, which develops and interprets the statutory law. It is also the source of common law, or case law, which is the law that develops from the decisions made by courts. Previous decisions are considered precedent and binding on all lower courts. In Latin this is called *stare decisis*, which means to stand by things decided or to adhere to decided cases.

Constitution and Bill of Rights

The Constitution and the Bill of Rights are two historical documents that guarantee certain fundamental freedoms to individuals. They affect the healthcare system by providing the fundamental rights to privacy, equal protection, and freedom of speech and religion (Box 1-2).

The United States has a two-court system: federal law and state law. The supreme law of the land is our Constitution, which establishes shared powers between federal and state governments. Cases in which the U.S. Constitution and federal statutes are violated or applied are heard in federal district courts (trial courts), district courts of

---

BOX 1-2
Amendments to the Constitution

Bill of Rights

Amendment 1—Freedoms, petitions, assembly
Amendment 2—Right to bear arms
Amendment 3—Quartering of soldiers
Amendment 4—Search and arrest
Amendment 5—Rights in criminal cases
Amendment 6—Right to a fair trial
Amendment 7—Rights in civil cases
Amendment 8—Bail, fines, punishment
Amendment 9—Rights retained by the People
Amendment 10—States' rights

Other Amendments

Amendment 11—Lawsuits against states

Amendment 12—Presidential elections
Amendment 13—Abolition of slavery
Amendment 14—Civil rights
Amendment 15—Black suffrage
Amendment 16—Income taxes
Amendment 17—Senatorial elections
Amendment 18—Prohibition of liquor
Amendment 19—Women's suffrage
Amendment 20—Terms of office
Amendment 21—Repeal of prohibition
Amendment 22—Term limits for the Presidency
Amendment 23—Washington, DC, suffrage
Amendment 24—Abolition of poll taxes
Amendment 25—Presidential succession
Amendment 26—18-year-old suffrage
Amendment 27—Congressional pay raises

BOX 1-3
Checks and Balances

Executive branch: President or Governor; can veto legislation and enforces the laws

Legislative branch: proposes and passes legislation; can override the President or governor

Judicial branch: interprets legislation; can overrule laws and actions of the executive branch

appeals, or the U.S. Supreme Court. When a suit is not connected in some way to federal constitutional issues, such as divorce or a traffic violation, it is tried in a state court. Each state has its own constitution that often mirrors the U.S. Constitution.

The constitutional basis for federal involvement in healthcare is found under the provision for the general welfare and regulation of interstate commerce. The states have the power to regulate healthcare through their police power to protect the health, safety, and welfare of their citizens. This includes the regulation of nurses, pharmacists, physicians, chiropractors, physical therapists, and other licensed healthcare providers.

Checks and Balances

Each branch of government serves as a check and balance for the other branches of government (Box 1-3). The legislature proposes and passes statutes and can override the veto of the President or Governor. The Governor or President can propose that legislative action be taken or veto legislation, appoint or nominate individuals to certain courts, and enforce the laws. The court interprets the laws and can declare laws that the legislature develops unconstitutional. This interaction provides the checks and balances for each branch.

The court also interprets regulations and their applications to individual cases, but not until all remedies provided by the regulations are exhausted. For example, the Board of Registration of Pharmacists and the employer of Brett, a pharmacist, accuse Brett of drug diversion. After a hearing, the board suspends Brett's license as a pharmacist. Brett may appeal the case to the court. However, if no hearing occurred, Brett could not appeal to the court, because he has not exhausted his remedies.

Common Law versus Civil Code

Finally, we should discuss two unique ways that laws can arise: common law versus civil code.

Common law develops from decisions previously made by courts, or precedents, and these are binding on all lower courts. In Latin this is called *stare decisis,* which means to stand by things decided or to adhere to decided cases. Common law originated from England with the Pilgrims and original settlers of the land. Since that time, each state's courts have made decisions regarding civil and criminal cases (Box 1-4). These legal principles were developed when the King pronounced rules on the basis of his divine right. Case decisions were accumulated and based on reason and justice. All the states, except Louisiana, have adopted the common law system. Because each state adopted different statutes and judicial interpretations, variations of the law exist among the states.

Only Louisiana, originally colonized by France, adopted a civil code based on the Napoleonic Code. The code is law created by the legislature rather than the judiciary.

BOX 1-4
Common Law Versus Civil Code

Common law: developed on a case-by-case basis from England when the king decided on the basis of his "divine right"
Civil code: developed from Roman law codified by the legislature

BOX 1-5
Civil Law versus Criminal Law

Civil law: case brought by an individual or entity against another individual or entity for harm based in tort, contract, labor, or privacy issues
Criminal law: case brought by the state or federal government for violation of written criminal code or statute

It is a comprehensive written set of rules and regulations rather than case-by-case analysis and interpretation of legal issues. It is based on Roman, Spanish, and French civil laws, not on English common law.

Types of Law

A common way to classify law is whether there is a civil wrong (often called a **tort**) that causes harm to a person or a person's property or a criminal wrong that violates criminal statutes (Box 1-5). Lawsuits against healthcare providers can be criminal or civil lawsuits. The distinction is the remedy or penalty, often called a *sanction*. The following sections take a closer look at the distinctions between these two types of law.

Criminal Law

Criminal law is concerned with violations against society based on the criminal statutes or code. The remedies in state or federal criminal cases are monetary fines, imprisonment, and death. Misdemeanors are lesser crimes punishable by (usually modest) fines

Relate to Practice
A patient is seen for an office visit and consents to the physician's removal of several skin lesions on the patient's arm. During the procedure, however, the physician does need to remove deeper tissue than he originally thought would be necessary to ensure that all margins are removed (in case the specimen is confirmed as malignant). The patient was not informed of the possible risks of scarring and is unhappy with complications of infection in the arm's healing because of the depth of the incision. The patient sues the physician.
1. Can the physician have any charges brought against him criminally?
2. How can a case like this be avoided?
3. What responsibility does a patient have in these instances?

BOX 1-6
Remedies

- *Civil remedies:* usually monetary award
- *Criminal remedies:*
  1. Misdemeanors: lesser fines and jail time of less than 1 year
  2. Felonies: major fines and jail time of more than 1 year, or the death penalty (in some states)
- *Administrative remedies:*
  1. Monetary fines
  2. Required education
  3. Loss of license to practice

established by the state and/or imprisonment of less than 1 year. Felonies are more serious crimes punishable by much larger fines and/or imprisonment for more than 1 year or, in some states, death. In many states, a felony conviction may be the grounds for revoking a license to practice in a healthcare field. A healthcare provider may be prosecuted criminally for practicing without a license, falsifying information in obtaining a license, or failing to provide life support for a patient. There are also the related felony charges of assault and battery. A patient who is treated without consent may file charges against the provider for assault and battery. Similarly, a patient who is detained without consent can file charges of false imprisonment. These are all criminal charges that could be filed against a healthcare provider.

Civil Law

Civil law encompasses various areas of law, including (but not limited to) contract issues, intentional torts, negligence, malpractice, labor, and privacy issues. Most cases against healthcare workers are for negligence or malpractice. Lawsuits against healthcare providers often include allegations of failures to provide care that meets the standard of care and result in harm or injuries to the patient. The remedies (Box 1-6) in civil law are almost exclusively monetary. The court cannot impose servitude or make the plaintiff whole again when the plaintiff has suffered such things as loss of a limb, pain, or emotional problems. The monetary award is an attempt to make the person "whole again." On rare occasions, the court may order a person to stop performing an act until a full hearing is held on an issue, to prevent harm from occurring that money cannot remedy.

Torts

The term tort comes from Latin, meaning to twist, be twisted, or to wrest aside. Tort is a private, civil, or constitutional wrong or injury, and not a breach of contract, for which the court provides a remedy for damages. There must always be a violation of some duty owed to the plaintiff, and generally such duty must arise by operation of law and not by mere agreement of the parties.

Negligence is a type of tort. It is the cornerstone of a malpractice case. Negligence does not require a specific plan to harm someone. There are four elements in a negligence action: duty, dereliction of duty, direct cause, and harm/damages (Box 1-7), which will be discussed in later chapters.

BOX 1-7
Elements of Negligence

Duty
Breach of duty
Direct cause (causal connection)
Damages/injuries

Malpractice requires proof of a breach of a standard of care, and the breach must cause damage or harm. Malpractice is a term used to describe the negligence of professionals, including healthcare providers. You will hear it most often in reference to nursing, medicine, healthcare, and law, although other professionals commit malpractice in their fields.

What If?

?

Facts: A 75-year-old patient at a licensed healthcare provider care center suffered from diabetes, dementia, coronary artery disease, and immobile decubitus ulcers (bedsores) and was unable to walk, talk, or feed herself.

Her physician prescribed a daily whirlpool bath as a medical treatment for the decubitus ulcers. The facility did not have a whirlpool so she was given a regular daily bath. A certified nursing assistant prepared a bath for the patient and placed her in hot water that was 138°F and that subsequently caused severe burns from which she died 3 days later.

A wrongful death action was brought. Parties settled before trial for $1.5 million.

1. Who will be named in this suit?
2. How could the patient's death have been prevented? How could a safer environment have been provided?
3. Define the four elements of neglect in this case.

Source: *Strine v. Commonwealth of Pennsylvania et al.,* 894 A.2d 733 (Pa. 2006).

The Court System

Now that we have an idea of the very basic categories of lawsuits a healthcare professional may most commonly experience, let us examine the usual sequence of events of a lawsuit—from filing through final appeal. This will give us an impression of the overall function of the U.S. court system. Both state and federal courts approximately follow the same three levels, dividing most cases into the following sequence: (1) trial courts, (2) appellate (appeals) courts, and (3) the state supreme court. Most medical malpractice suits, excluding issues such as Medicare fraud, are tried in the state courts because they usually violate state regulations. For that reason, we will first examine the typical state court system.

State Trial Courts

Primarily, the local courts usually address crimes and civil cases that do not exceed a certain minor monetary sum established by the legislature. These often involve no jury

> **BOX 1-8**
> **Jurisdiction**
>
> *In personam:* The court has jurisdiction or control over the person.
> *In rem:* The court has jurisdiction or control over the thing or property.

and are handled quickly. The next level of court is a court with general jurisdiction, referred to as a major trial court with fairly broad powers. It is in this court that medical malpractice, elder abuse, negligence, major crimes, and other civil wrongs are tried. In some states, specific courts may be specialized, handling a specific type of case exclusively, such as family or probate cases, juvenile cases, or housing or land issues. These specialized courts are limited in their jurisdiction to only specific types of cases.

To try a specific case, the court must have jurisdiction (Box 1-8) over the case. Jurisdiction can be *in personam* or *in rem. In personam* jurisdiction means the court has jurisdiction over the person. For example, the major trial courts' jurisdiction is based on county or parish lines or other such divisions. This means that a case must be tried in the county or parish in which the incident leading to a suit occurred. The plaintiff may have the option of presenting the case in his or her own county or parish, depending on the rules of procedure for that state. Also, some cases may only be pursued in federal courts (e.g., bankruptcy, admiralty). In certain instances, the plaintiff may have to file a case where the defendant lives, such as in cases involving collection of money owed.

In rem jurisdiction means the court has jurisdiction over the property or thing itself rather than over the people involved. The court determines the right to the specific property, which is binding usually against the whole world, not just the parties involved.

In addition, filing a suit must be timely; that is, it must be filed within the statute of limitations—a claim must be filed within a specific amount of time of discovering that a wrong has been committed. Statutes of limitations vary not only from state to state but also from one kind of offense to another.

Next, as a case is prepared for trial, responsibility rests on the plaintiff to prove his or her case, as opposed to the defendant. An exception to this would be if the case is decided by a judge (pretrial) to be *res ipsa loquitur,* which means "the thing speaks for itself." This would have to be established by the plaintiff pretrial and ruled on by a judge in most states. *Res ipsa loquitur* means that there is clear evidence of negligence and there was no possible way that the patient (plaintiff) could have affected a different outcome or contributed to the damages or injury. It also indicates that there is clear proof that the defendant had the responsibility (duty) to the patient and that the injury would not and could not have occurred without the negligence of the defendant.

The name of a case indicates who is suing whom. The person or entity bringing the suit is called the plaintiff. For example, the patient who brings a complaint against the hospital, healthcare provider, or facility is the plaintiff. The person or entity who is sued and defending against the allegations is the defendant. The plaintiff is listed first in the caption and the defendant is listed after the versus *(v.),* such as *Alexis and Brett Kyle v. Alexandra Hospital.* See Box 1-9 for an outline of how cases are named.

Pretrial Discovery
Before trial, both sides have strategies for gathering information in preparation for the trial; this is called the discovery process. These discovery strategies include the following:

BOX 1-9
How to Read a Case Citation

Plaintiff's name v. Defendant's name, Volume number, Name of reporter, Series number, Page number (Court name, Year)

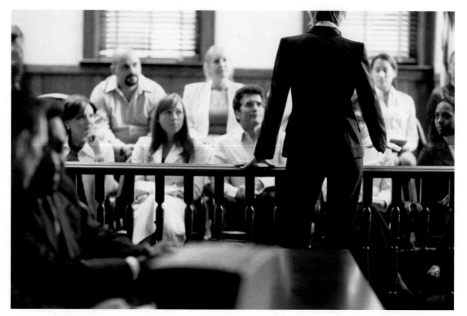

Figure 1-2 The facts, as found by a jury or judge, cannot be appealed.

1. **Interrogatories** are written questions that must be answered in writing under oath, sent by one party to another. They are part of the discovery process to prepare for mediation, settlement, and trial.
2. **Requests for production of documents** are submitted to the opposing party to produce specified documents or items that are pertinent to the issues of the case such as medical records or policies and procedures.
3. **Admissions of fact** ask the opposing party (in writing) to admit or deny any material fact or the authenticity of documents to be introduced into evidence at trial.

Courts of Appeals

Once a trial is completed or a case is final in the court of general jurisdiction, or in one of the specific courts, a case may be appealed to a higher court, usually called an appeals court or **appellate court**. There are both state and federal appellate courts. An appeal may only raise an issue of law. The facts, as found by the jury or the judge, cannot be appealed (Figure 1-2). If the appeals court decides a case and no further appeal is taken, the appellate decision is binding on all lower courts in the state.

State Supreme Courts

From the state appeals court, an appeal may be taken to the top court of the state, usually called the **state supreme court**. Again, only issues of law can be appealed. The

---

BOX 1-10
The U.S. Federal Courts

- U.S. Supreme Court
- U.S. court of appeals (appellate court)
  - 12 Regional circuit courts of appeals
  - 1 U.S. court of appeals for the federal circuit
- U.S. district courts (trial courts)
  - 94 Judicial districts
  - U.S. bankruptcy court

---

state supreme court does not act on most cases, and the parties have no recourse for further review unless a **writ of certiorari** is filed with the U.S. Supreme Court and the Court chooses to hear the case. The ruling by the U.S. Supreme Court is binding on all state courts.

Federal District Court System

Before we continue to examine the role of the supreme court in this trial sequence, now is a good time to briefly compare the federal and state court systems. Needless to say, the sequence is nearly identical because state court systems are modeled, for the most part, after the federal court system:

Cases concerning federal, Constitutional law are filed and tried in federal district court. There are 94 judicial districts organized into 12 regional circuits. Each circuit has a U.S. court of appeals (Box 1-10). In the federal court system, if a case that has been decided in a district court undergoes appeal, the appeal is next decided in the regional circuit court of appeals. Following the regional circuit court, the only appeal for a federal case is through the U.S. Supreme Court, which may or may not agree to review the case.

The U.S. Supreme Court

The Chief Justices choose the cases that the **U.S. Supreme Court** hears. The party appealing either a federal circuit court's decision or a state supreme court's decision with a federal question files a petition called a writ of certiorari. The U.S. Supreme Court chooses very few cases to hear. As with appeals coming from state supreme courts, only issues of law can be appealed, not issues of fact, and, as with the state systems, the state supreme court does not act on most cases.

Those cases that are chosen must involve a question of substantial importance. For example, the case *Roe v. Wade* posed the question as to whether the constitutional rights of women and of developing embryos and fetuses require that abortion be legal for some portion of the pregnancy. Once the U.S. Supreme Court decides a case, it is binding on all state and federal courts.

What If?

A nursing assistant's job requires him to change positions and take vital signs on all his patients every 4 hours. Today, however, his workload almost doubled since he worked with a new patient and did not have time to do these tasks for the last patient on his list. To try to keep up with everything, he just copied the vital signs taken 4 hours earlier and falsified that he turned the patient.

1. Could the nursing assistant be held legally responsible for this action?
2. What are some possible legal repercussions if this patient suffers damage from the nursing assistant's failure to act in this case?

What If?

A facility's policies and procedures and/or physician's order state that the patient's vital signs must be taken every 4 hours. Is it a form of negligence if you decide not to take vital signs because the patient is sleeping?

Conclusion

This chapter is merely a brief introduction to the terms and concepts found in this text. Many of the concepts in this chapter will be defined and explored in more detail in subsequent chapters. The idea of this chapter is to provide an overview of some of the technical concepts of the laws and the processes of law and to begin to define how the laws directly affect healthcare professionals.

Chapter Review Questions

1. One of the four elements of negligence is
   A. dereliction of duty.
   B. deliberate act.
   C. the defendant.
   D. executive branch.

2. The statute of limitations refers to
   A. the amount of time it takes to go to trial.
   B. the amount of time someone has to file a lawsuit.
   C. the sentencing given in a lawsuit.
   D. All the above

3. The civil cases seen in courts are suits that involve
   A. criminal acts.
   B. relationships.
   C. employer-related cases.
   D. real estate only.

4. The term _____ means that a particular legal issue was settled in another similar case, setting a precedent.
   A. *res ipsa loquitur*
   B. malpractice
   C. tort
   D. *stare decisis*

5. *In rem* jurisdiction means the court has jurisdiction over
   A. civil law cases.
   B. malpractice cases.
   C. property.
   D. appeals only.

Self-Reflection Questions

1. Discuss the reasons and goals of the law.
2. Discuss how the law changes.
3. Discuss how the various sources of law might interact or affect one another.
4. Describe the differences between civil, criminal, and administrative law.

Internet Activities

1. Go to the law library or use the Internet to obtain a copy of an actual case in your area of practice. (Use recommended websites.)
2. Investigate the medical practice acts for your state online and review procedures for licensing.

Additional Resources

www.findlaw.com

www.lexisone.com or www.lexisnexis.com/community/portal/ (To research cases a fee is charged. Other information from the site is still free.)

www.usa.gov

www.definitions.uslegal.com

www.uscourts.gov

Chapter 2

The Basics of Ethics

Jeanne McTeigue

KEY TERMS

Accreditation Process of officially recognizing a person or organization for meeting the standards in an area based on preestablished industry criteria.

Applied ethics Application of moral principles and standards to organizations of individuals.

Bioethicists Specialists who study the ethical dilemmas resulting from advances in medical research and in science.

Bioethics Ethical dilemmas and issues that arise attributable to advances in medicine.

Code of ethics Standards of behavior, initiated by an employer or organization, defining the acceptable conduct of its members/employees (also called code of conduct).

Duty-based ethics (deontology) Philosophy of ethics that focuses on performing one's duty to a group, individual, or organization.

Ethics Branch of philosophy that relates to morals and moral principles.

Integrity Unwavering adherence to an individual's values and principles with dedication to high standards.

Justice-based ethics Ethical philosophy based on all individuals having equal rights.

Medical practice acts Laws defined by each of the states that regulate the licensing and medical laws for that state and define the scope of practice for licensed and unlicensed individuals in the healthcare field.

Morals Standards of right and wrong. Moral values that govern behavior and beliefs based on principles of right and wrong. The norms of measuring right from wrong.

Rights-based ethics Philosophy of ethics based on theory of the rights of each individual (autonomy).

Scope of practice Officially sanctioned description of the specific procedures, actions, and processes that are permitted for a licensed or nonlicensed professional; based on the specific state's laws for education and experience requirements, plus demonstrated competency. Established by the state's laws, licensing board, and/or agency regulations.

Standards of practice Basic skill and care expected of healthcare professionals in the same or similar branch of medicine; based on what another medical professional would deem to be "appropriate" in similar circumstances (also known as standards of care).

Tolerance Respect for others whose beliefs, practices, race, religions, or customs may differ from one's own.

Utilitarianism Ethical theory based on the greatest good for the greatest number (also known as cost/benefit analysis).

Values Principles that individuals choose to follow in their lives.

Virtue-based ethics Ethical theory or philosophy that relies on the principle that individuals share and will hold as their governing principle the values of moral behavior and character.

CHAPTER OBJECTIVES

1. Define *ethics* and explain the various layers of ethics.
2. Outline the specific forms for applied codes of ethics used in the medical field.
3. Describe instances of subjectivity as related to ethics.
4. Define and explain *bioethics*.
5. Examine the importance of ethics in healthcare.
6. Relate specific ethical theories to healthcare situations.
7. Apply one of the ethical decision-making models to a specific ethical healthcare dilemma.
8. Explain the function of an ethics committee.
9. Discuss the concepts of risk management and quality assurance.

Introduction

The study of ethics and bioethics is a necessary part of preparing for the medical field. Individuals employed by healthcare organizations often face dilemmas that the general population does not encounter; these unique situations require critical thinking, the ability to observe situations objectively, and sound decision-making strategies.

Ultimately, most allied health professionals are accountable to a physician or hospital, but this does not exclude them from responsibility. Understanding the law and standards of practice helps allied health professionals make sound decisions in ethical situations.

What Are Ethics?

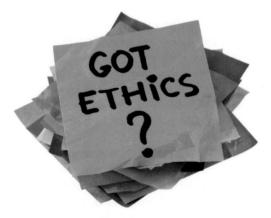

Ethics encompasses several different facets. First, as a branch of philosophy, ethics studies the values that influence human behavior, tying our actions to a sense of right and wrong. A second aspect is an individual's ethics; this refers to one person's moral principles—the values that govern a single person's decisions with a goal of maintaining one's integrity or conscience. These may include, but certainly are not limited to, honesty, fidelity, gentleness, fairness, compassion, responsibility, humility, and respect for life. Finally, group ethics is a system of principles and rules of conduct accepted by a group or culture. For instance, medical ethics will be of particular interest to readers of this book.

How do you know when you are facing an ethical dilemma? First, your conscience will usually be affected. If you have a quandary that makes you lose sleep or feel uncomfortable, it is more than likely an ethical dilemma. Your next question in such a situation is to ask yourself whether the issue is one of ethics or personal values. There may be circumstances where a proposed action is not necessarily against a code of ethics, but it may be an integrity issue for you personally. Our personal beliefs and values may have higher or different standards than those outlined in a particular code of ethics. For instance, one person may be strongly opposed to abortion, but the facility where the person is employed may legally perform abortions. This would then become a personal dilemma for that individual and not a dilemma for the facility.

We will examine more closely the ways that these layers, or categories, of ethics overlap and contribute to one another. We have just established, for example, that values are the principles that an individual chooses to follow in life. Although these may be personal values, they are also the qualities that drive most ethical behavioral models for groups. Individually, a person may value loyalty or privacy as well as freedom. For a group, the code of ethics would mirror these values and require that all employees or individuals involved in that group adhere to the principles prescribed in that organization's code of ethics.

Discussion
Of the following qualities, which do you think is the most important virtue in the medical field?

- Honesty
- Fidelity
- Integrity
- Justice
- Respect
- Empathy
- Sympathy
- Responsibility
- Hard work
- Fairness
- Sanctity of life
- Gentleness
- Compassion
- Humility

Codes of Ethics

Applied ethics relates to the ethical policies that are applied to organizations. All organizations have a code of ethics policy or a code of conduct policy that they expect their employees to follow. Usually a healthcare organization's code of ethics will include statements regarding the treatment and care of the patient as the most important priority, most importantly treating all patients with dignity and respect. These in turn dictate such standards as guarding and respecting patient confidentiality. Violation of the code of ethics in most organizations incurs sanctions or corrective action and/or removal of membership.

Medical Codes of Ethics

Ethics, as with laws, provides us with a "yardstick" by which we can measure behavior. Beginning with Hippocrates ("the father of medicine"), we have a documented medical code of ethics, and his Hippocratic Oath has been pledged by medical professionals over the centuries. Building on this, the American Medical Association (AMA) has designed a more encompassing, more contemporary code of medical ethics for physicians. This was enacted initially by the organization in 1847 and was most recently updated in 2001. As medicine and the medical profession grow and change, this code is continually reviewed and refined.

Using this model, all areas of the allied health field and most organizations have developed their own codes of ethics, such as the American Association of Medical Assistants (AAMA), the American Academy of Professional Coders (AAPC), nursing associations, hospitals, and large healthcare facilities and organizations. (See Additional Resources for further information on examples of the Hippocratic Oath and codes of ethics.)

Tolerance

Finally, while we apply both personal ethics and a group code of ethics in the healthcare workplace, we must learn to practice tolerance, for the sake of our own professionalism. Tolerance is respect for others whose beliefs, practices, religions, or customs may differ from our own. Tolerance must be practiced by all healthcare providers in all fields. We do not have to agree with or condone the behaviors, beliefs, or practices of another individual but we can never pass judgment by our actions or words against another person. Understanding that all people have the right to their own beliefs and practices and that our diversity as a social community is to be celebrated and not lamented will help the allied health professional to view others with respect and to treat others with dignity and compassion.

Medical Ethics

In the medical field the applied code of ethics serves as the basis for the more specific standards of practice that are adopted and accepted for that area of medicine. These codes can take several forms.

Standards of Practice

Also known as standards of care, each major allied health and medical specialty has established its own set of ethical and professional principles in a standards of practice document. This official document establishes basic requirements for skill and care commonly used and expected of the healthcare professionals of that same or similar branch of medicine, and thus establishes what another medical professional would deem to be "appropriate" in similar circumstances. For example, it would be a standard of practice principle that all physicians would obtain an updated history and physical form for a patient they had not seen in a number of years, to update their medical history. This is a practice that would commonly be practiced or expected. Another example is a principle stating that a surgeon must review and obtain written consent for surgical procedures, outlining all the common risks.

Medical Practice Acts

Almost all healthcare professionals—such as physicians, pharmacists, social workers, dietitians, physical therapists, emergency medical technicians (EMTs), medical assistants, and others—have prescribed scope of practice guidelines that are determined by medical practice acts established in each state. These laws establish and govern licensing boards and regulations that describe requirements for education and training, and define the scope of practice for the individual practitioner in a given field. The scope of practice in each case is the document that defines the procedures, actions, and processes that are permitted for licensed and nonlicensed individuals in that field. The scope is limited by the provisions of the law required for education, experience, and demonstrated competency. Working within the guidelines of the scope of practice can protect the professional from any personal liability. Conversely, if a medical professional acts outside the scope of practice for his or her field, that professional would be considered medically liable if any personal harm occurred.

Ethics and the Challenges of Subjectivity

Ethics can be a gray area and may seem to be subjective (that is—changeable, depending on a person's perspective) because of different circumstances and the particular events involved. For that reason, it is our duty as allied health professionals to act with conscious consideration of the consequences and ramifications of our choices, always weighing our actions and reactions using critical thinking skills to determine the proper course of action.

Repeated Wrongs

One challenge of subjectivity is that individuals have the ability for self-deception, convincing themselves that their wrong actions are acceptable. Time and repetition enhance this skewed vision of ethics. Over time, a repeated wrong action becomes less troublesome to the individual's conscience. For example, an employee takes sample drugs from the cabinet without the physician's approval. There are no consequences. Subsequently, it becomes commonplace for this individual (and possibly witnesses) to believe it is acceptable to take drugs from the sample supply whenever the drug representative provides more samples. The individual believes his or her action is acceptable even though he or she is aware that the purpose of those samples is to provide patients with a temporary supply of the medication in order to test the efficacy and possible side effects of the drug. Employee use of those samples should only be granted with the provider's permission.

Ignoring a Witnessed Wrong

A second problem with subjectivity is that of ignoring inappropriate behavior. Individuals may witness or be aware of an inappropriate action, even a serious crime, and can sometimes convince themselves they are innocent of ongoing misconduct because they are not the perpetrator. This, similar to the ability to feel less accountable that may occur from repeated acts of transgression, is nevertheless a moral failure or an eroding of one's ethics. It can also be illegal to keep such secrets.

What If?
You witness a coworker openly treating a patient disrespectfully because of his or her personal opinion of the patient. If the patient feels that he or she is being treated in a disrespectful or discriminating fashion, the patient could very well make a complaint or claim against the provider. What would you do if you witnessed this happening?

Once you are aware of a transgression, it is your responsibility to act on it. Your own liability rests in the fact that once you are aware of an offense and fail to prevent it, you are just as guilty of the violation. In the case of fraud, you could be held financially and criminally liable.

> ### ? What If?
> What would you do if you observed any of the following situations?
> 1. You discover another employee is embezzling money from the practice.
> 2. You find that another employee is falsifying records and not truly performing the vital signs for patients.
> 3. You realize that the practice is billing for services on a patient that were not performed.

Subjectivity and the Needs Hierarchy

You may be aware of Abraham Maslow's Hierarchy of Needs pyramid (Figure 2-1). This theory asserts that human beings have needs that must be satisfied in a specific order for us to self-actualize—that is, to become our highest, most moral and ethical version of ourselves. From basic needs to the highest need, these needs fall into the following order (Maslow, 1954, p. 236):

1. Need for basic sources of life: water, food, sleep, shelter
2. Need to be in a safe environment
3. Need to belong and to be loved
4. Need to feel responsible and valued (self-esteem)
5. Need to contribute, to find personal growth and fulfillment (self-actualization)

Obviously, while we may recognize early in life that stealing, for example, is wrong, it is easier to adhere to this principle if you are financially successful in life than it is if you have a child who needs food or water to survive. Although such extreme disparities do not typically arise for healthcare professionals in the United States, we may encounter patients, even patients who have committed crimes, who are on quite a different level of need than we are and whose value differences may reflect that disparity.

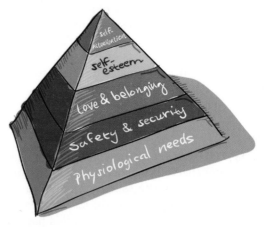

Figure 2-1 Maslow's Hierarchy of Needs.

Bioethics

Another ethics challenge in the medical field occurs when personal values and professional goals—even humanitarian goals—conflict with one another or become, at the least, uncomfortable. For example, the study of bioethics, or biomedical ethics, is the study of ethical dilemmas that arise as medicine advances. The men and women who study these issues are called bioethicists. Examples of bioethical issues include stem cell research, genetic engineering, and the Human Genome Project. We will look closer at some of these issues later in the chapter, when we turn our attention to medical ethics specifically.

Ethics versus Law

Most would agree that illegal acts are most likely unethical, but there are many unethical behaviors and/or actions that are not necessarily illegal.

Because law and ethics are so closely interrelated, medical professionals, and all choosing careers in the allied healthcare field, need to have a thorough understanding of both of these in order to protect themselves, their employers, and their patients. This chapter discusses the elements of ethics, ethical models, and theories on handling ethical dilemmas.

As allied health professionals, it is vital that we understand all legal and ethical ramifications of our actions and behaviors. The factors involved in the Discussion example should be based on medical necessity guidelines solely and not on reimbursement. The provider must always present the patient with the ideal options of treatment and diagnosis for optimal medical treatment and these options should not be regulated or dictated by insurance or reimbursement protocols. This example also offers insight into interpersonal medical ethics because it deals with ethical communication and interaction of the healthcare providers.

Discussion

Should a healthcare professional treat a patient differently based on their insurance coverage?

1. How would or could that impact the patient?
2. What, if any, legal complications could occur? Malpractice?
3. What should a medical assistant do if witnessing this?

Relate to Practice

A medical assistant is working in a family practice clinic when a patient requires an immunization. The physician takes the medical assistant aside and explains that it is a particularly busy day, especially since the nurse has called in sick. She asks the medical assistant to administer the injection so she can proceed to the next patient. The medical assistant explains that it is not within the scope of practice in his state for him to administer an injection. The physician insists, saying she will take that responsibility. What should the medical assistant do?

Relate to Practice

It had only been a week ago that Janie had been so excited about being hired for her first job as a medical assistant at the women's wellness clinic in town. During her interview, the office manager had asked her several questions pertaining to injection skills and her ability to handle upset or angry patients. Janie felt that she had given suitable answers to all the interviewer's questions. When asked if Janie had any questions, she had asked about several policies that the clinic had in place for their employees, such as workplace attire, company sick days, and weekend work schedules.

Now, just 1 week into her new job, Janie feels completely unprepared to handle the situation that now confronts her. To her dismay, she learns that the clinic routinely performs legal abortions. A devout Catholic, Janie had not thought about the clinic performing abortions nor the fact that, as an employee, she would be called upon to be a participant in the process. What should Janie have done differently? What should she do now?

Medical Etiquette

Medical etiquette is a matter or courtesy and manners in relationship to ways the medical professionals handle each other and ways the patients are addressed, especially those with disabilities or mental disorders. In terms of professionalism and customer service, medical etiquette concerns how physicians and staff handle their patients. The standards of professionalism expected in the medical field need to include showing patients respect and tolerance no matter the circumstances. As healthcare providers and workers, we must always bear in mind that most patients either are not well or may be facing stressful challenges and may not be themselves; these patients may not always be polite or may not even be very cooperative. The focus should be on the patient's well-being and most healthcare workers need to remember "it's not personal." Handling mentally ill, belligerent, or uncooperative patients can pose extra dilemmas, such as preventing an escalation of their anxiety or anger. Using a calm, but not patronizing, tone and showing respect for them as individuals can make all the difference. Exhibiting professionalism and maintaining composure in these instances are essential. Many specialized facilities, such as those that work with mental health patients, offer special training or workshops in handling particularly challenging situations in a safe, but professional, manner.

Ethical Decision Making

Now we will turn our attention to how ethical principles for governing groups have been used over the years to establish theories and models for ethical decision making. As we examine both the theories and the models, as well as the basic ethical group principles upon which they are founded, we will explore these in terms of the medical and healthcare professions specifically.

Principles of Healthcare Ethics

We will begin with the building blocks of ethical medical practice: the ethical group principles on which the theories and models that help us in our daily work are built.

The principles of group ethics are both the basis and the goals established for all subsequent ethical theories developed. Although many principles can apply to healthcare, such as respect, fidelity, and veracity, a few are of special importance in the medical field and thus are the foundation for ethical theories embraced by allied health professionals. We will examine the following four of these foundational principles, emphasized by the AMA:

1. Beneficence: The principle of doing the "most good" and/or benefiting the largest number (principle behind utilitarianism).
2. Nonmalfeasance (least harm): Similar to the principle of beneficence except the focus is to do the least amount of harm to the least amount of people (seen in the Hippocratic Oath: "first do no harm").
3. Autonomy: The principle that acknowledges that individuals have free will to make decisions about themselves and the paths that they wish to pursue. However, this can be contrary to what is best for a patient's health.
4. Justice: The principle that prescribes that ethics should be based on what is consistent and fair to all involved. Uses logic as it basis.

Discussion
Give an example of medical dilemmas affected by one or more medical principles of healthcare ethics as listed in this chapter.

Ethical Theories

Most ethical theories are based on group ethics principles such as those previously discussed. Philosophers have developed these theories over the years to explore their effects on individual and group behavior. Although there are several ethics theories, particularly because these affect group behavior and group governance, most fall into one of the following categories: utilitarianism (a type of teleology), duty-based ethics (deontology), rights-based ethics, and virtue-based ethics. We will examine each of these next, especially as they apply to medical ethics specifically.

Ethical Theories

Utilitarianism	The greatest good for the greatest number
Duty-based ethics or deontology	The obligation of the individual to fulfill his or her responsibilities
Rights-based ethics	Based on an individual's rights
Justice-based ethics	No special advantages or disadvantages to certain individuals
Virtue-based ethics	Actions are based on the individual's character

Utilitarianism (Teleology)

One of the most commonly known ethical theories is utilitarianism. This theory is a type of consequence-focused theory known as teleology. Utilitarianism bases the decision making on the greatest good for the greatest number. This theory is based either on the greatest benefit to the general population as a whole (or the best total outcome) or on the final consequences and not on the process. It is also referred to as "the ends justifying the means." It therefore does not always take into account the "means" but instead the general final outcome: What will benefit the greatest number of people? For example, this theory may be used in determining the use of funds, organ donations, and other resources available. Utilitarianism is implemented to determine the most efficient use of resources (the best value for the least number of resources) and looks beyond individual impact to overall benefits.

This is also known as cost/benefit analysis because it takes into consideration the cost of resources versus the overall benefit.

Medical Application

Suppose a practice is interested in purchasing new equipment. A first step might be to perform a prospective audit to determine the projected earnings of owning that equipment and the number of their patients who would benefit from the use of that equipment, and then these results would be compared with the cost of the equipment. For example, a neurology practice wants to purchase an electromyogram (EMG; used for nerve conduction testing) machine that costs slightly more than $20,000 dollars. If they charged the insurance companies approximately $1000 for each testing and they had at most 20 patients whom they had been referring elsewhere for this test, then it would be cost-effective and profitable for the practice to make that investment.

What If?

1. There was a shortage of flu vaccines in a given year; what would the utilitarian model recommend be done?
2. There were several patients who needed a liver transplant and only one liver was available; what criteria would be used to determine who gets the liver donation?

Duty-Based Ethics or Deontology

This theory is based on the duty of an individual to a society, group, or organization and focuses solely on the obligation of the individual to perform his or her responsibility, no matter what the circumstances. The general principles include impartial thinking with respect to individuals as not being the "ends to justify a means" and absolute rules that should be obeyed. In other words, it is the duty of an individual to adhere to universal rules and regulations, regardless of circumstances.

Medical Application

If it is a nurse's duty to take the vital signs of each of her patients every 4 hours, she must do so regardless of the situation. The problem with this theory is that not all "duties" are defined that simply; it does not take into account the conflicting duties that may arise. For instance, if the same nurse is taking vital signs on her patients every 4 hours and one patient has cardiac arrest and the nurse has to perform cardiopulmonary resuscitation, the nurse misses the 4-hour timeframe and has violated her duty to take the vital signs timely for the rest of the patients. This theory is based on impartial judgment and does not take into consideration the consequences. Thus, as we see, it can cause an additional dilemma if the duties are conflicting.

Rights-Based Ethics

This theory is based on the individual's rights. The emphasis is on the specific person and does not always take the consequences of the general population into consideration, asserting instead that those rights should be upheld in spite of the circumstances. For example, the right of free speech and the right to bear arms have been developed and upheld by the U.S. Constitution. It takes only the individual's rights into consideration and therefore it can conflict when the rights of a society or an organization are in jeopardy (e.g., upholding an individual's right to bear arms versus the need for gun control regulations to keep guns out of the hands of irresponsible, dangerous, or unstable individuals). Under this principle, the individual's rights must be respected, even though this may be contrary to society's rights as a whole. If misused, this could lead to individual gain without regard for damage or harm that can be caused to others.

Medical Application

Patients sometimes have religious beliefs that contradict those of their family members or other patients; an example would be medical needs for certain treatments such as blood transfusions. If the patient is the child or dependent of such individuals, and that child's life is in danger, the physician has an ethical dilemma. Whose rights should be honored, especially if the child is not able to express his or her own preferences?

 Discussion

In the medical field, an individual has the right of freedom of religion, yet it may be contraindicated for the effective treatment of the patient. How does a physician handle a case in which a child needs a blood transfusion to save his life yet the parents' religious beliefs do not allow blood transfusions? Does the physician using the rights-based ethical model respect the religious beliefs of the parents and allow the child to die? Or does the physician respect the child's right to life, despite parental beliefs?

Justice-Based Ethics

This theory is based on the ideal that "justice is blind"—that is, all individuals should be treated with impartiality and there should be no advantages or disadvantages to individuals. The philosopher John Rawls believed that the principles of this theory would prevent unfairness and injustice under social contracts, such as the distribution of organ donations. One individual should not have a greater chance over another. For example, a person with greater financial means should not have more power than a person with less financial means (Figure 2-2).

Medical Application

Consider the case for the ideal of socialized medicine. Under this system, individuals are all treated equally and theoretically would not be able to gain advantages based on income, age, race, or other factors. This theory is considered to be a democratic one based on the fairness and justice for all and the "veil of ignorance"—that justice is impartial and blind. The controversy arises in that some feel that it is unfair for the healthy to help pay for the support of the unhealthy or that it is more "democratic" or fair that advantages are "earned" and justified.

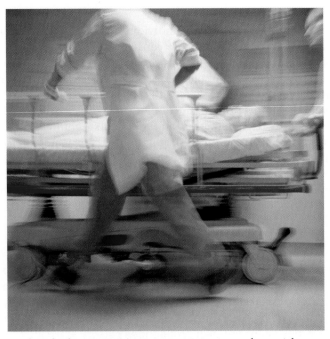

Figure 2-2 Justice-based ethics is meant to prevent injustice under social contracts, such as the distribution of organ donations. One individual should not have a greater advantage over another.

Virtue-Based Ethics

This theory places an emphasis on the character traits and qualities of individuals, such as honesty, integrity, and industriousness. Its focus is the individual striving for a better life—according to Aristotle's theory that the goal of our lives is to find happiness and that this is not achieved solely by our prosperity in life but instead by our character.

Medical Application

While her colleagues vote to strike for a fairer pay-scale, one that is more commensurate with the rest of the economy (and with salaries at other similar institutions), a nurse at an eldercare facility may be uninterested in striking because she believes that her most important values are her innate characteristics of compassion and patience. Therefore she finds happiness in caring for her patients and feels she needs nothing else. Virtue-based ethics theory does not take consequences into account. It is also flawed by operating on the assumption that everyone's virtues and actions are universal. However, because this is usually not the case, some persons may be treated unfairly.

Relate to Practice

An EMT is loyal to his company because of his own virtues and set of values. The employer treats this EMT unfairly by not bothering to reward this employee with raises, increased benefits, fairness in assigning days off, or other recognition, or worse by mistreating that employee. Who bears responsibility? Who is wrong: the employer for unfair manipulation or the employee for loyalty?

Ethical Decision-Making Models

After developing ethics theories based on basic principles, philosophers have taken the next step by developing theoretical models to be tested and/or used as guideposts for application by individuals and groups faced with ethical dilemmas. The ethical theory applied depends on the circumstances and events involved. In that way, what starts as a theory may become the basis for many of our regulations and laws.

First, we will look at a basic model for making ethical business decisions. Asking yourself the following questions (from the Blanchard-Peale ethical decision-making model [Peale & Blanchard, 1988, p. 27]) can help you determine whether you are making an ethical management choice or decision:

1. Is it legal?
2. Is it balanced?
3. How does it make me feel?

When facing a difficult choice, keep in mind that no ethical decision should be based on emotions. Ethical dilemmas should be faced and handled with logic and facts, weighing the alternatives and the consequences, and keeping an objective mind, as we will see in the models that follow. These two models are used by decision makers to evaluate ethical dilemmas properly.

The Seven-Step Decision-Making Model

There are many different versions of this model but all have the same intention: to determine the facts of the event or dilemma and to use this tool to assess all the possible options in a thorough and objective manner.

1. Determine all the facts of the situation—what, when, where, who, and why.
2. Determine the exact ethical issue involved.
3. Determine the rules, laws, principles, or values that are involved.
4. List ALL possible options or courses of action.
5. Determine all the advantages and disadvantages of each option.
6. Determine all the possible consequences and who would be affected by the options.
7. Determine which decision is best and act on that decision.

In some situations and at certain institutions, these steps may all be done by one individual or by a group of individuals. There may be an ethics committee that would evaluate the situation, and one member may have just one of these steps to complete, and then all individuals involved would meet to determine the best course of action. This may be accomplished in collaboration with a *risk management team* or a *quality assurance team.*

Dr. Bernard Lo Clinical Model

The second model is one developed by Dr. Bernard Lo and relates directly to the medical field. His model is designed to take into consideration the patient's point of view as well as that of the provider:

1. Gather information—Patient's mental status, comorbidities, views of the other healthcare providers for the patient, and other issues that might complicate the patient's case.

2. Clarify the ethical issue—What is the defined ethical issue involved? What principles should be employed and what are the ramifications of the courses of care possible?

3. Resolve the dilemma—List alternatives available and discuss with all healthcare providers for the patient; negotiate the best possible options. If the patient is mentally competent, make the patient part of this process also.

Medical Etiquette in Decision Making

Medical etiquette is not a model, but it is its own unique challenge because it deals with the customs and manners used as they relate to the medical field. As a general rule of etiquette, for instance, a front desk receptionist would not leave a physician waiting on the phone or sitting in the waiting room for a long period of time. These customs have changed over the years and do vary according to the circumstances, but generally they are respectful manners because they pertain to handling of other individuals in the medical profession.

Ethics Committees and Quality Assurance

Ethics Committees

Most very large medical facilities (particularly hospitals) assemble an active group of employees or administrators to become part of the ethics committee for that organization. These persons involved do not generally see or speak with the patients themselves but focus solely on the facts involved in the situation. This helps them make ethical determinations on the issues or cases presented to them on the basis of logic and on the codes and standards, as opposed to emotions.

Accreditation

As we have seen earlier, establishing and maintaining appropriate standards of care is an essential part of ensuring that we provide universally ethical facilities. One way we keep standards high is accreditation—the process of officially recognizing a person or organization for meeting the standards in an area based on preestablished industry criteria. Many facilities and organizations maintain voluntary participation with accreditation organizations, who routinely examine the organization or facility to verify (as an objective party) that the standards of care and procedures of the organizations are in compliance. Typically for hospitals, this accreditation organization would be The Joint Commission (TJC). (A full listing of accrediting organizations can be found at www.anab.org.)

Risk Management and Quality Assurance Programs

All medical facilities and practices should have a form of either and/or both of these programs. These committees are formed to evaluate and ideally prevent situations that arise and cause ethical dilemmas. They evaluate patient satisfaction, patient complaints, and treatment outcomes. In the medical billing and coding side of the field, they evaluate and audit records for completeness and accuracy in prevention of fraud and billing abuse. These committees concern themselves with prevention and improvement of policies and recommend and monitor actions that noncompliant healthcare facilities can take for improvement. The facility's own risk management team also evaluates staff for prevention of injuries on the job.

Discussion
Is it right that a committee would have the right to life-and-death decision making for patients and yet not even interview these patients?

Conclusion

All members of the medical profession, in whatever capacity they are working, must understand their responsibility to themselves, their employers, and their patients—to uphold the highest standards of ethical behavior and professionalism. Also, we live in a litigious society, an unfortunate reality, and we must always consider the consequences of our deeds and behaviors. Using the described models and thinking critically to determine our best courses of action will alleviate a considerable degree of emotional stress and aid the healthcare professional in making the best possible decisions.

Chapter Review Questions

1. An example of utilitarianism would be the
   A. decision of which patients should receive immunizations if supplies are limited.
   B. decision of employees' rights in a work resolution.
   C. decision of what was fair in a given work resolution case.
   D. decision in a malpractice suit of responsibility in the case.

2. The movement of etiquette-based medical practice is concerned with
   A. moral principles.
   B. standards of care.
   C. courteous, nonpreferential treatment of patients.
   D. moral dilemmas.

3. What does an ethics committee handle?
   A. Decisions in possible violations of codes of ethics
   B. Decisions of workplace rights
   C. Decisions of hiring practices
   D. Legal decisions on scope of practice

4. What are values?
   A. Principles by which an individual chooses to live
   B. Moral guidelines for the workplace
   C. Manners and etiquette
   D. Workplace hiring guidelines

5. What is autonomy?
   A. Individual's right to make decisions for one's own life
   B. Group ethics guideline
   C. Accreditation
   D. Risk management principle

Self-Reflection Questions

1. What kinds of ethical situations would be particularly challenging or difficult for me to encounter?
2. What would I do if my best friend became my coworker and I witnessed him/her doing something unethical at work?
3. Which of the principles of ethics is the most important to me?
4. Which of the ethical theories do I find most agreeable?
5. Using an ethical dilemma scenario you create, follow one of the two decision-making models discussed in this chapter to determine the best course of action.

Internet Activities

1. Research several different code of ethics models that apply to your field and develop your own model.
2. Research online the different versions of the Hippocratic Oath and discuss why there are different versions.

Additional Resources

www.ncbi.nlm.nih.gov/pubmed/8044100

www.ama-assn.org

www.ama-assn.org/ama/pub/physician-resources/medical-ethics/code-medical-ethics/history-ama-ethics.page?

www.cms.gov

www.aama.com

www.onlineethics.org

www.pbs.org/wgbh/nova/body/hippocratic-oath-today.html

www.aapc.com

www.ascensionhealth.org/components/com_filesandlinks/uploads/96_clinical_ethics.pdf

www.anab.org

www.corrections.com/news/article/23352-ethical-leadership-part-2

www.history-ama-ethics.page

www.ama.assn.org/ama/pub/physician-resources/medical-ethics/code-medical-ethics/history-ama-ethics.page

http://dgim.ucsf.edu/about/lo.html

www.kenblanchard.com

Bibliography

Lo B: *Resolving ethical dilemmas: a guide for clinicians*, ed 4, Philadelphia, 2009, Lippincott Williams & Wilkins.

Maslow A: *Motivation and personality*, New York, 1954, Harper, p 236. ISBN 0-06-041987-3.

Peale NV, Blanchard K: *The power of ethical management*, ed 1, New York, 1988, William Morrow, p 27.

Rathburn KC, Richards EC: Professional courtesy, *Missouri Med* 95:18-20, 1998. Accessed at http://biotech.law.lsu.edu/Articles/Professional_Courtesy.html.

Chapter 3

Ethical and Bioethical Issues

Jeanne McTeigue

KEY TERMS

Advance directives (living wills) Means by which a patient can self-determine his or her wishes to use any artificial means to continue life if he or she is unable to communicate them in the future. These can include healthcare proxies, living wills, and durable power of attorney declarations.

Artificial insemination (AI) Injection of seminal fluid into the female vagina, which contains male sperm from a husband, partner, or other donor, to aid in conception.

Chromosomes Threadlike structures in the center of the cell (nucleus) that transmit the genetic information about the person.

Clone Duplicate cell reproduced artificially from a natural, original single cell.

Control group Group of subjects in a research study who do not receive any treatment or, in some cases, are given a placebo. In testing, it is the principle of the constant that remains the same to evaluate the changes of a given experiment.

Do not resuscitate (DNR) Form completed by patients to indicate in advance that no means should be used to regain function of cardiopulmonary processes when these functions cease (e.g., cardiopulmonary resuscitation).

Euthanasia Termination of a life to eliminate pain and suffering related to a terminal illness, usually performed by giving a drug or agent to induce the termination of bodily functions. Also known as assisted suicide.

Fertilization Assistance in conception, most commonly performed either as artificial insemination or as in vitro fertilization to produce pregnancy.

Gene therapy Process of splicing or infusing genes to replace malfunctioning genes. Alteration of the DNA of body cells to control production of a particular substance.

Hospice Organization or program involving a multidisciplinary group of medical professionals available to aid in support of the terminally ill and their families.

Human Genome Project Medical research program, sponsored by the federal government, established to map and sequence the number of genes that are within the 23 pairs of chromosomes (i.e., the 46 chromosomes) with the goal of advanced life-saving or disease-preventing treatments.

In vitro fertilization Process to assist in conception by harvesting ovum from a female and combining it with the male's sperm outside of the uterus and then implanting the fertilized embryo back into the female's uterus.

Nontherapeutic research Medical research in which the test subjects are not necessarily suffering from a disease or the particular disease that the study is researching, and therefore the subjects are not receiving a direct medical benefit from participating in the study.

Palliative care Literally meaning to ease or comfort; the care provided to terminally ill patients to alleviate symptoms and discomfort suffered while dying.

Placebo Nontherapeutic drug or agent given to a control group. (Commonly referred to as a "sugar pill.")

Stem cells Cells of the body that can control the production of specialized cells by becoming other types of cells as needed during growth or healing.

Sterilization Any procedure performed to permanently prevent reproduction.

Therapeutic research Medical research performed on chronically or terminally ill patients who may benefit from the agent being tested.

Uniform Determination of Death Act (UDDA) Model state legislation that has since been adopted by most U.S. states and is intended "to provide a comprehensive and medically sound basis for determining death in all situations."

CHAPTER OBJECTIVES

1. Define the term *bioethics*.
2. List at least three key biomedical issues associated with medical research.
3. Identify two methods of artificial conception and discuss associated key ethical questions.
4. Describe ethical considerations for healthcare professionals in issues of genetic testing and stem cell research.
5. Describe ethical questions related to death and dying.
6. Explain the function of an advance directive, a living will, and a DNR form.
7. Outline basic concerns in ethical issues raised by both proponents and opponents of healthcare reform.

Introduction

Currently, much of our media exposure and knowledge concerning bioethics seems like science fiction. In fact, debates over controversies in bioethics often parallel science fiction discussions. So, what exactly is bioethics? Bioethics is a field of study (and debate) that examines ethical questions raised not only in medicine but also in biotechnology and discusses the ways that new scientific advances affect—and have the potential to affect—our lives. Bioethics embraces issues such as gene splicing and manipulation, genetic code interpretation, cloning, in vitro fertilization, and stem cell research. Some of the issues discussed in this chapter would not have been considered a decade or two ago. However, bioethics also embraces issues that have existed for some time, including abortion, death and dying, and scientific research as it affects subjects, patients, and families.

Bioethics

Bioethics can be defined as the field of study examining the ethical dilemmas surrounding advances in bioscience and in diagnostic and treatment procedures, as well as ethical issues involving medical research. First of all, advanced research carries with it not only important discoveries but also challenges to the rights and privacy of its subjects. Second, although it is very true that medical advances bring hope for recovery from diseases that would automatically have been fatal in the past, the discouraging side of these advances is that the rights of individuals are sometimes threatened as a result. In addition, sometimes patients have to choose between experimental or potentially life-saving treatments that may prolong life but deprive good quality of life. Faced with such grim options, patients may make end-of-life choices that may personally conflict with those of their practitioners. Finally, the healthcare system forces ethics decisions on us every day because we must take into consideration that an estimated 46 million Americans are without health insurance and if the costs of treatment for the uninsured are not covered some of these patients will die (Bialik, 2009, p. A12).

Medical Research

We will first discuss bioethical issues surrounding medical research. Although there can be many ethical challenges in research, most often these issues raise the following types of questions:

- In a study, how much should research subjects be told about test results, especially if informing the patient may skew the accuracy or "blind" aspect of the study?
- What is our responsibility if a patient-subject is adversely affected by a study? Also, what is our obligation to inform other patients?
- Is it unfair to conduct research on animals, because they have no voice or choice? If so, what restrictions should we have on the procedures we subject to animals used in research labs?
- Next, how do we choose which research results to promote when funding is limited—those that will save the lives of a small number of patients or those that may effect only moderate improvements but could positively affect a larger number of people?
- Finally, advances in science have raised new ethical questions for all of us: for instance, is it ethical to save lives by harvesting stem cells from embryos? Is it less of an issue if the embryos were frozen and slated for disposal anyway? In addition, should we be allowed to modify an individual's genes or stem cells, even to avoid future disease?

Of course, we cannot follow-up on all of these research issues, but we can focus on a few that have resulted in a significant impact.

Sometimes violations of ethics in medical research go so far as to become criminal actions. The case provided in the Discussion box would certainly violate the laws describing the rights of patients in most states today, but historically perhaps the most noteworthy examples were the inhumane experimentation performed on individuals in German concentration camps during World War II. Victims were brutalized in bizarre ways under the guise of "medical research" until the War ended and the details of the experiments were uncovered during trials of Nazi war criminals. As a result of these trials, codes of ethics were developed in the international medical community, and now today many of the current codes of ethics are still based on the principles outlined in the Nuremberg Code.

However, what about genuine research? When do ethical lines become blurred in this case? The atrocities inflicted on the victims of the WWII concentration camps represent a deviant distortion of the scientific processes, and obviously the main goal of *ethical* medical research is to restore or prevent illness and to reduce deaths and disabilities caused by diseases. We will next discuss the elements of any responsible medical research project.

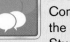

Discussion

Consider the very famous case of the Tuskegee Syphilis Research Study. In 1929 the health departments of six different states, in conjunction with the U.S. Health Service department, conducted an experiment in order to attempt to control venereal disease. Statistical reports had shown that between the years of 1930 and 1932 in Macon County, Alabama, 84% of the population was black males and 40% of all males were infected with syphilis. At that time the method of treatment for the disease was an injection of mercury and other toxic chemicals. Some patients were cured by this method, while others became more ill or died. Patients who were not treated with the injections were found to live for several decades. Some untreated patients suffered from organic brain syndromes and later developed dementia.

After funding for the research was exhausted during the Great Depression, the researchers conducting the Tuskegee Study decided to further examine the disease to determine its long-term effects. They selected 600 men, 400 of whom had been infected with syphilis before the study and 200 who were not infected. The 200 uninfected men were labeled the *control group*. During the study, in order to promote patient cooperation, the infected men were told that some invasive procedures (e.g., lumbar punctures, or spinal taps) were part of the treatment when actually these procedures were only diagnostic; in addition, the subjects were never informed of the study's objectives. Any of the 200 subjects who contracted syphilis while in the study was simply transferred to the other group and subjected to the study's

procedures without treatment; in addition, some of the subjects were never informed that they had contracted the disease. None of these subjects were ever given any informed consent.

The study continued well into the 1940s when the discovery of penicillin occurred, and yet these subjects were denied treatment with the antibiotic that would have cured them. The antibiotic not only was withheld but also the study was continued, even though there was no need to further study "untreated" patients with this disease because a cure had been found. It was not until a researcher who worked for the Public Health Service alerted the media, after imploring the researchers to cease their research, that the study finally ended in the 1960s. By this time, the Centers for Disease Control and Prevention was supervising the project in Atlanta, Georgia.

In 1973 the surviving patients received an "out-of-court" settlement of $37,500 for the infected men and $16,000 for the men in the noninfected group. The families of the men who had passed away received $15,000 and the men who died in the noninfected group's families received only $5000.

- What kind of a difference would it have made in these men's lives if they had participated with informed consent?
- Why should the studies have been discontinued after the discovery of penicillin?
- In the previous chapter we learned that ethical medical behavior should always be governed by the principles of autonomy, beneficence, and nonmaleficence. How did this study measure up to these three principles?
- How fair do you think the settlements were?

Informed Consent and Blind Studies

Clearly, in order to maintain the objectivity of any research using human subjects, some information must be withheld for the trial to be successful. Also, no medical research is risk free—there is always an element of risk involved, but the patients or subjects of the study should be fully informed of the risks and give full written consent. This is an example of the utilitarian theory of reasoning—that is, the greatest good for the greatest number would outweigh the risks involved for the study's subjects, particularly if they will not benefit or if they suffer side effects or health risks from the research. For instance,

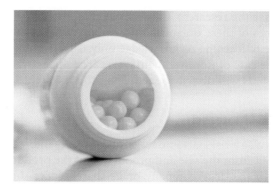

Figure 3-1 In a blind study, patients may receive no drug (the control group), the new trial drug, or a placebo.

suppose a study is testing the efficacy of a new pharmaceutical agent for Parkinson's disease. This is considered a therapeutic research trial because the subjects might benefit directly from the treatment or drug being tested. Patients involved in the trial would be informed that they may be receiving no drug (the control group), the new trial drug, or a placebo (Figure 3-1). We call this a blind study, because the patients do not know whether they are receiving the placebo or the new agent. This ensures that the subjects will not have any preconceptions of the effects of the drug and helps them be more objective.

However, this is where the ethical dilemma develops: In therapeutic trials like our theoretical one, participants have usually reached a point at which the illness or disease has been unchanged by any other type of treatment option, and indeed for some the study may be a last resort for a cure or symptomatic relief. Unfortunately, if they are given the placebo, patients who need treatment are not actually receiving any medication for a significant period of time.

Once a drug or treatment is past the initial research phase and has been approved for use by the U.S. Food and Drug Administration (FDA), it is distributed for use by the public. Unfortunately, because the needs of the drug are immediate, long-term effects of the drug or treatment may not be fully identified before it is approved for use.

All medical research studies must be closely monitored and must meet guidelines and approval from the American Medical Association (AMA) and the Department of Health and Human Resources (DHHS). If a hospital or federally funded facility is sponsoring the research, they must also establish an institutional review board (IRB)

What If?

The daughter of a former patient contacts the hospital where her father died to say that she saw a commercial on TV from a law firm asking the general public if they have ever had a reaction, a side effect, or a family member who has died because of the adverse effect of the drug her father was taking at the time of his death. Records show that he too suffered from the adverse effect and that it is possible, though not conclusive, that this may have led to his death. She decides to sue the hospital for negligence.

Question: Should anyone be able to sue for an adverse reaction to a medication or treatment? If not, who should regulate the cases that may be considered for litigation?

to oversee the research. Those conducting the study must abide by the standards and guidelines of these organizations, and no persons should be put at significant risk for the sake of learning or knowledge only. This is not a valid reason to risk human life.

In the case of nontherapeutic research this is even more vital, because none of the participants will directly benefit from the research.

Conflict of Interest

There is also a risk, in some cases, of conflict of interest. For example, if a drug company will profit from the sale and production of the product being tested, then no one affiliated with the drug company or its shareholders should participate in any way. The same should be said in the case of studies involving medical diagnosis and the study of diseases and causes. If a physician is part of a statistical tracking process for his or her own medical theory, it is too difficult to remain objective toward proving that theory correct, and the evidence the physician provides might be compromised by his or her own subjective influence in the study.

 Discussion

Wakefield Study
In 1998 Andrew Wakefield, MD, published the results of a study in *The Lancet*. Dr. Wakefield and other researchers studied 12 patients and found a link between gastrointestinal illness and autism. The study connected the illness with the MMR (measles, mumps, and rubella) vaccines that these patients were given and suggested that the gastrointestinal illness caused by the vaccine had resulted in the onset of autism for these 12 patients. The study was only conducted on 12 subjects, but it was considered valid and the number of immunizations in countries in Europe and the United States plummeted because of parents' fears that the immunization would cause autism.
What is the problem with this study?

Ethical Issues in Reproductive Medicine

Contraception and Sterilization Issues

The issues that arise in regard to sterilization and reproduction are a broad category. In this section we will cover some of the main topics that have become ethical and bioethical areas of concern and debate. In light of the advances in medicine, many of these are current and newly developing issues of concern and as we continue to advance, the ethical and bioethical issues will, no doubt, also increase.

Voluntary Sterilization

Some patients seek surgical procedures to voluntarily alter their ability to reproduce. Female sterilization methods (e.g., Essure) and surgeries (e.g., tubal ligation) aim to prevent the ovum from leaving the fallopian tubes and sperm from fertilizing the ovum. Males may opt to undergo a vasectomy, which isolates the vas deferens to prevent sperm from entering the seminal fluid. Patients may choose these procedures for many reasons; reasons may be economical (e.g., the patient cannot afford children) or therapeutic (e.g., the patient is at risk because of conditions such as cancer), and some patients simple do not wish to reproduce. In all cases, the providers must use careful screening and detail issues of consent to ensure patients understand that undergoing such procedures is intended to be a permanent decision. Some providers will not perform these procedures on anyone younger than 30 years of age and prefer that the patient has already reproduced before making this choice. In most states, the law forbids the sterilization of any minor, except in extremely rare cases involving a court order.

Involuntary Sterilization

In the past, these procedures were performed on patients who were deemed to be unfit mentally and/or who had a severe genetic disorder, to prevent them from passing on the disease or illness genetically. Although many people feel that this is an unethical procedure, it was fairly commonly done and until recently was mandated in many states. More recently, especially in light of proof that not all severe mental illness is hereditary, this practice has become less frequent. In most states the procedure would be ordered only if the case was presented that the patient themself would be in danger or would endanger the unborn child. This raises ethical and legal challenges such as designating who would make the determination of when to require an individual to be sterilized involuntarily.

Contraception and Abortion

Religious beliefs are major contributors to the ethical and legal questions surrounding these two issues and encompass debate on everything from the many different types of contraception to the "morning after pill" to the options of abortion versus adoption for pregnancies conceived outside a parent's willingness or ability to keep a child.

Because of their own ethical standards and also in light of the large controversy surrounding the subject, many healthcare providers will not perform voluntary abortions. If an abortion is performed in the early weeks of pregnancy, the patient should not suffer any long-term effects of the procedure, but in the cases of late-term abortions, many complicating factors become involved. The following key questions remain in debates on abortion: "When does human life begin?" "Does it begin upon conception when the genetic DNA is initiated, or does it begin in the embryo or fetus, or not until the child is born?" The arguments continue.

> ## Discussion
> Before abortion was legal, desperate women tried illegal services, usually engaging in unsterile, dangerous procedures to end pregnancies; it was not unusual for both the woman and her fetus to die. Conversely, now that abortion is legal, some women abuse abortion rights by using it as a form of birth control rather than as a last measure. Which is worse? Do you feel it should be legal?

Conception Issues

Bioethical issues are also raised when addressing assisted or artificial conception. These can take several forms, ranging from artificial insemination (AI) and in vitro fertilization to surrogate motherhood.

Artificial Insemination

This procedure is commonly used for patients who are unable to conceive a child by natural means and involves implanting male sperm into the woman's vagina to aid in conception. The sperm may originate from the woman's partner, from the woman's husband, or from a donor. This is rarely an issue when the procedure is performed for a husband and wife or for a couple and the donor is known. However, there are instances when situations can alter one individual's consent, causing ethical and legal dilemmas.

For example, some cases have involved women using frozen sperm collected from a husband before his death in order to conceive a child. In many states, this raises legal questions regarding the rights that the child has to the father's estate, pension, or social security benefits, for example. Another dilemma occurs when donor sperm is neither that of the spouse nor that of the partner, and full consent was not obtained by the partner for the implantation. The partner could then legally refuse to provide care and support for the child. Alternatively, relationship ethics could come into play if the resultant pregnancy leads the noncooperating partner to suspect the woman of adultery instead of undergoing the medical procedure. These issues are often further complicated by the fact that many states have not yet established laws in this area so there may not be clear-cut regulations regarding donor sperm. From the standpoint of the healthcare provider, informed consent from both the patient and the partner is the best protection.

Discussion

In addition to these challenges just discussed, more complications can arise later as the child grows. Choose one of the following questions for reflection and discussion:

- If donor sperm is used, will the partner treat the child the same as he or she would a biological child?
- Is a donor's hereditary information available to a child so that when the child matures he or she might discover his or her genetic background? Should the child and the donor have the option of meeting (as in the movie *The Kids Are All Right*)?
- What if the donor sperm was not obtained from a legitimate sperm bank?
- What if the child has unknown siblings from the donor that would make it unwise for him or her to marry or date, but the child is unaware of this fact?

In Vitro Fertilization

Another procedure to assist couples in conception involves the harvesting of the woman's ova and the combination of these ova with the partner's sperm cells to then be grown outside of the womb; the fertilized ova are then later implanted into the uterus. This procedure—in vitro fertilization—is now so commonly accepted that many insurance companies currently reimburse the costs for this procedure (Figure 3-2).

Ethical choices still exist, however. First, of course, the patient and partner must be completely informed and each must provide full informed consent of the procedures to be done in combining the ovum and sperm and in harvesting the eggs. They should also be aware that unused ovum and sperm as well as unused fertilized eggs (embryos) are usually destroyed. This may be an ethical problem for some patients, which, of course, then leads to the debate of when human life begins. Some believe that life begins the moment that the sperm and ovum are joined and the fertilization process begins; others argue that life begins once the fertilized egg becomes an embryo at 8 to 14 days; and still others contend that life does not begin until the organs begin to form and the embryo becomes a fetus between the eighth and ninth weeks. Then there are some people who argue that a life does not begin until the child is born.

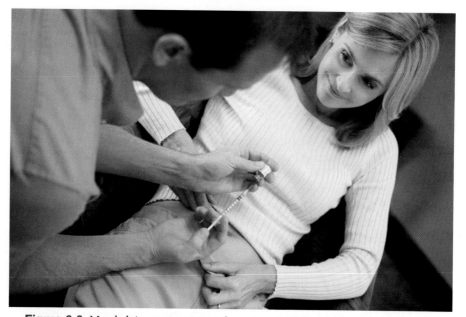

Figure 3-2 Man helping woman inject drugs in preparation for in vitro fertilization.

Relate to Practice

Most states vary but all have laws dictating what they consider the legal life of an unborn child. Maria, a nurse in a psychiatric facility, is 12 weeks' pregnant. She has just arrived at work and has been on the floor making medication rounds for 20 minutes when a patient, hiding behind his door, leaps on her, punches her, knocks her to the floor, and kicks her in an attempt to leave the facility. Maria is injured and hospitalized. Examinations and tests prove that her unborn child was killed in utero during the assault. Aside from the death of her unborn child, Maria herself should make a complete recovery, both from the assault and from the miscarriage. Her physician is confident she will be able to have other children. Can the person who committed the assault also be charged with murder?

Surrogate Motherhood

In surrogate motherhood, a woman agrees to have a child for another married heterosexual couple or for a homosexual couple. This may mean carrying the fertilized embryo of a married couple for a female unable to carry the child, or it may involve using the *in vitro method* to impregnate the surrogate, in cases in which the female is unable to produce ova so the surrogate's ovum or another donor's ovum is used. In each of these types of surrogate motherhood, the sperm may or may not be obtained from the couple. This, of course, has led to a number of legal and ethical issues, especially in custody battles.

Consider the famous custody case of Baby M. Eventually the case was heard by the New Jersey Supreme Court, and custody of the child was given to the Sterns, a couple who had contracted with Mary Beth Whitehead to surrogate the child. This legal battle had begun when the surrogate mother, Mary Beth Whitehead, threatened suicide just after giving up Baby M. following the birth of Baby M. in March of 1986. The Supreme

Court ruled on this case, granting parental rights to the biological mother despite the contract established with the Sterns, but it awarded physical custody to the Sterns, because this was deemed to be in the best interest of the child, with the biological mother awarded visitation (*New York Times*, 1988, in re Baby M., 537 A.2d 1227, 109 NJ 396 [1988]).

What If?

A couple struggles for several years with infertility and finally feel they have found the perfect solution: they hire a surrogate. They meet with the young woman and like her immediately. As they talk, there is an instant connection, and both parties sign a contract. Upon becoming pregnant, the young woman agrees that this child will be the couple's child. In return, they provide for her during her pregnancy, cover all medical expenses, and are supportive of her emotionally, attending all prenatal exams and even birthing classes. When the baby is born, the young surrogate mother is emotional, but gives the infant to the couple as agreed. They are thrilled and grateful. Unfortunately, 2 months later, they receive a letter from an attorney claiming that the surrogate mother has changed her mind. She wants the child.

Should a surrogate mother be allowed to change her mind once a child is born? If so, under what circumstances? Would you answer differently depending on whose ovum and sperm were used? Should the child's age make a difference?

Genetic Testing and Counseling

The concept behind the screening of parents genetically is to avoid reproduction when the possibility of transmitting a terminal or disabling disease exists. These diseases, such as phenylketonuria (PKU), sickle cell anemia, Down syndrome, cystic fibrosis, and Tay-Sachs disease, just to name a few, can cause infantile death if not treated immediately and/or can cause a lifetime of disability. Parents can theoretically make rational decisions to conceive a child on the basis of genetic possibilities through screening. Unfortunately, some testing cannot be done until the fetus is developing, and then the decision to continue the pregnancy full term or to terminate the pregnancy becomes a more ethical issue. Most hospitals now do screening of newborn infants for PKU and other disorders so that the infant can be treated immediately—in cases of PKU with special diet requirements—and this would prevent the death of the infant.

Ethical Issues in Biomedical Advances and Genetics Research

Gene splicing, or gene therapy, and stem cell research are genetic advances that could potentially rid the population of a significant number of diseases and prolong life. These issues, of course, have both supporters and detractors. Many feel that the knowledge, and therefore the power of this knowledge, could lead to distorted use of this information by individuals who have a perverted or self-serving agenda.

Gene research and gene therapy concentrate on finding ways to manipulate our existing genes to identify those that cause specific diseases and conditions. The hope is that someday we can manipulate or eradicate genes that contribute to serious diseases. By contrast, stem cell research and therapy focus on duplicating or growing stem cells from human embryos and other tissues to—as with genes—pinpoint those that either promote or eradicate serious diseases or conditions. In some types of cancer, we have already been able to use stem cells to extend the patient's life significantly.

The Human Genome Project

Beginning in the 1990s, the Human Genome Project was started to enable researchers to map the genetic code of the DNA found on each cell and the 24 pairs of chromosomes that define individuals. The purpose of this research is to identify and hopefully treat and/or prevent diseases and disorders that are genetically transmitted, such as sickle cell anemia and cystic fibrosis. Ideally, knowing the patient would be predisposed to certain diagnoses, the patient can be treated before the symptomatic problems and thus prevent serious health issues. The advances of this global research have identified many connections between illness and genetic predisposition. For instance, we now know that if a patient has allergies and chronic bronchitis, this is genetically transmitted in the same gene that transmits eczema and asthma.

As it advances genetic engineering is focused on preventing the transmission of these diseases by correcting the genetic code in the current chromosomes and then the subsequent transmission, theoretically, would be corrected for future generations. This could lead to the elimination of diseases such as colon cancer, other cancers, and Alzheimer's disease.

Stem Cell Research

Stem cells are unique cells that have the ability to divide indefinitely and to develop into many different types of cells, particularly during early life when growth and development are underway. Their function is to aid healing by providing essential replacements. For example, a single stem cell, on division, has the potential to either remain a stem cell or become almost any other kind of specialized cell, such as a brain cell or red blood cell. In studying these cells, researchers found a way to obtain stem cells from human embryos and then grow these cells in laboratory conditions. These are called *human embryonic stem cells*. Because these embryos were created through in vitro fertilization in lab conditions for research purposes and were then destroyed (with donor consent) when no longer needed, their use became highly controversial.

The good news is that in 2006 researchers learned how to alter specialized cells in adults to create a new type of stem cell, called *induced pluripotent stem cells (iPSCs)*. Even so, controversy remains. Stem cells have the potential to treat, and even heal, many diseases, but the ethics involved in obtaining and using these cells will be ongoing for quite some time.

Discussion

Where should genetic engineering end? Through genetic testing and engineering, the cloning process began. The medical issue of "playing God" is of course the controversy that is prevalent. Would it be ethical, for instance, to **clone** a loved one or a lost child?

Ethical Issues in Death and Dying

Ethical issues in death and dying will be covered in detail in Chapter 10, but a brief overview of the types of ethical issues encountered is appropriate here.

Decisions to Prolong Life

No one likes to think about it, of course, but dying is a natural part of life. Conversely, we all pursue healthcare for ourselves and those we care about because we would like to live, and have those we love live, for as long as possible. However, how do we define really living, and what represents enough quality of life to make that feel worthwhile? The answer to this question is highly complex and individualistic.

Although death is inevitable for everyone, advances in medicine have enabled people to overcome a number of diseases. For example, suppose a patient has suffered from severe hypothermia: visible signs of breathing may be absent and there is barely a palpable pulse, but with the body in that state, the individual may indeed still be alive and can be revived with few or no lingering effects. As a matter of fact, some hospitals use artificially induced hypothermia to treat a patient and avoid the death of that patient.

Other medical advances may not cure a dying patient, but they may at least retard both the process and the side effects—and thus allow a patient who is essentially dying to live much longer than previously seen. For example, organ transplants, cancer treatment options, and advances in the treatment of heart disease have extended many lives. A patient may be considered dead when heart and lung function cease, but the use of CPR (cardiopulmonary resuscitation) can regain that function. Conversely, a patient may have full cardiac and cardiopulmonary function and yet suffer "brain death" when the brain ceases to function, leaving the patient comatose and nonresponsive. In these events, life-support systems may be implemented, such as ventilators and feeding tubes, to continue the body's functions for the patient.

If a patient is an organ donor, the body must have sustained oxygen available to the vital organs for them to be harvested and used for organ donation. In some cases, therefore, a patient may be clinically dead but yet have the body maintained until the harvesting of the organs can be completed.

So what happens when it is possible to extend someone's life, but the level of comfort, quality, and "fully living" comes into question? There are many controversial and ethical dilemmas surrounding these possible scenarios. The question of when exactly death occurs is as controversial as the question of when life begins. The issue of "quality of life" adds another layer, because no two members of one family may answer this in quite the same way, and when healthcare providers' own beliefs are brought into the mix, the end-of-life decisions for one single patient can become a complicated ethical debate.

Palliative and Hospice Care

The term **palliative care** comes from the Latin root that means *to ease* as in the cases of terminally ill patients. When there is no chance of regaining health and the illness is inevitably going to cause the patient's death, measures are taken to ease the suffering associated with the death process. Through medications and other means, the care of workers from hospice and other agencies helps to make the death process as painless and comfortable as possible for these individuals.

Hospice care also provides emotional support to the families as well during the dying process. The family's care is provided by a multidisciplinary team of nurses, physicians, and even counseling and spiritual support services to both the patient and the family.

Advance Directives and Living Wills

Increasingly more individuals are preparing documents called **advance directives** so that their loved ones will not have to make the critical decisions for them in case of

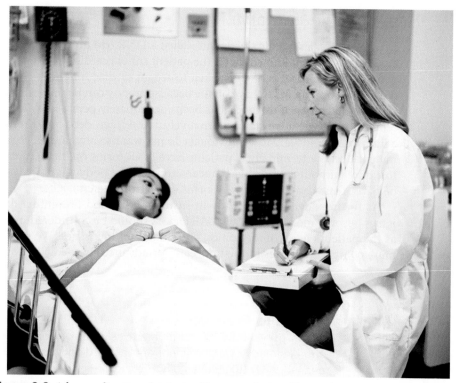

Figure 3-3 Advance directives let the healthcare professional know the patient's wishes when the patient is no longer able to communicate.

illness or accident. In 1980 the American Medical Association along with the American Bar Association and the American Academy of Neurology, as well as other organizations, developed and approved the Uniform Determination of Death Act (UDDA). This Act states that when a patient has irreversibly lost function of the entire brain (including the brain stem) and/or the circulatory and respiratory systems, they are considered to be dead. Advance directives let the healthcare professional know the patient's wishes when the patient is no longer able to communicate (Figure 3-3). The use of a living will, healthcare proxies, and a durable power of attorney also allows patients to make their wishes known ahead of time.

Of course, this is less likely to cause controversy if such documents are in place and recognized before it is time to make life-preserving decisions. In the landmark, ground-breaking, Karen Ann Quinlan case, the patient was automatically placed on a ventilator and given an NG (nasogastric) tube for feeding. In this case, the patient had become comatose after use of prescription drugs and alcohol. Once the patient was declared to be in a permanent vegetative state, the parents petitioned the courts to have these measures discontinued. The court eventually ruled that the ventilator could be discontinued. In this particular case, Karen lived for another 10 years before dying in 1985, but never regained consciousness. She was indeed able to breathe on her own but still was receiving the feedings via the NG tube. There were many debates in the media about the quality of her life. If this patient had a living will, the measures taken would not have been started. Greater ethical difficulties develop once these measures have been taken and then later requested by families to be discontinued. Clearly, the withholding of life-sustaining means is much less complicated than the removing of life-sustaining machinery after any of these means have been initiated.

Do Not Resuscitate (DNR)

In some states, a separate document, called a DNR (do not resuscitate) order, enables a patient to make it known that if the patient suffers cardiopulmonary death, he or she will not want measures of CPR taken to regain cardiac function. This is an important document for patients to have on file because a body can be revived with the following possible outcomes: if the body has been inadequately perfused by oxygen, it could be reduced to a vegetative state; alternatively, the oxygen debt could result in the loss of a limb or appendage. Most individuals do not want to remain in a vegetative state, and many elderly or terminally ill patients have DNR forms on file so that they may be left to expire without extraordinary means to keep the body alive. DNR orders may also be part of an advance directive. Forms differ from state to state.

As further advances are made in sustaining life and preventing death, the ethical issues become more complicated. All factors should be considered in these cases, such as the patient's age, comorbidities, and quality of life issues. We will continue to see more complicated cases in the future as our advances in medicine continue.

Relate to Practice

When 59-year-old Elizabeth T arrives in the emergency department, she is already cyanotic (blue) and all cardiopulmonary functions have ceased. After 20 minutes of CPR and life-saving measures, the patient is revived and placed on a ventilator. Since the physicians cannot yet assess whether the patient will regain brain function, the family is informed that the patient will most likely, if surviving the event at all, be left in a vegetative state. Should the family opt to have life-sustaining measures stopped?

Euthanasia

When does quality of life become the issue? In cases of terminal illness, should the patient be allowed assisted suicide or just the termination of artificial means to sustain life? The autonomy of our patients and their rights and control over their own lives, versus the duty of the medical team to preserve life, comes into question. At this point, the issue of euthanasia can become a factor. End-of-life cases have generally taken two routes: (1) actively assisting in a suicide, or euthanasia, and (2) simply withdrawing medical intervention for a patient. Many would argue that these two processes are vastly different and that withdrawing care or intervention is far different than actually causing the death of an individual. Others feel that it is simply a matter of allowing a patient who is dying to have autonomy over the method of death—just as patients are allowed to select their own treatment options after being fully informed.

At the time of this publication, it is illegal to assist in a suicide in a majority of U.S. states. Under very specific circumstances, in some states if at least two medical professionals affirm that a patient is terminally ill but of sound mind and not just depressed over the medical circumstances, that patient may be assisted in pharmaceutical suicide. However, these states are in the minority, and almost universally the debate remains on whether or not assisted suicide is murder.

It is a difficult situation for a terminally ill patient to face the stark reality of their prognosis. The medical and ethical issues around death and dying become increasingly more intricate as we advance in the ability to both prolong life and seek to grant patients autonomy over their own bodies. There are no easy answers.

What If?

A patient is diagnosed with early-stage Alzheimer's disease and she finds her son and daughter disagreeing on who should provide her care. What if she disagrees with both their ideas? What should she do to prepare for the time when she will no longer be able to make her own healthcare decisions?

Ethics in Healthcare Systems and Healthcare Reform

Healthcare Systems

Medical necessity should dictate the care of all patients. This is to say that the correct treatment of a given condition in the proper setting should be the course taken by any healthcare provider. What is in the best interest of the patient's welfare and health should always be the main factor in deciding how to treat a patient. Unfortunately, because of the changes in healthcare, the litigious nature of our society, and the fear of malpractice, this is not what determines all patients' treatment plans.

The facts of the matter are that it is the physician's duty to present to their patients the diagnosis, prognosis, and any or all treatment options. The patient, on the other hand, usually has insurance coverage that dictates its own medical necessity guidelines and restrictions on what it will reimburse for certain diagnoses and treatments. This causes major ethical dilemmas for healthcare providers.

Patients today are very accustomed to limited out-of-pocket expenses and are often not able to or not inclined to want to assume the expense that would be necessary for many procedures and treatments, including expensive medications. As insurance companies determine what treatments and pharmaceuticals they will cover, the decision is based on cost and profitability from their standpoint and is not always in the patient's best interest, especially in light of expensive medical advances in treatments and procedures available such as stem cell and gene therapy.

In the United States, insurance companies have become the dominating factor in most patients' treatments and options for treatments. They have determined the payment a healthcare provider can receive for given services since the healthcare provider needs to agree with the predetermined fee schedule for that insurance company or choose not to see patients with that coverage. This has become a serious ethical and moral issue for providers. A documentary film called *The Vanishing Oath,* by Crash Cart Productions, addresses the issues facing physicians in light of the ability to treat patients fully in the current model of healthcare.

Relate to Practice

During an office visit, Mr. H, who smokes cigarettes, is diagnosed with bronchitis. His physician wants to prescribe Levaquin because this is usually the best antibiotic treatment, and it is especially most effective for smokers with bronchitis. However, the physician knows that most insurance companies will not cover this expensive antibiotic. What should the physician do?

Healthcare Reform

The major controversy surrounding healthcare reform could be debated in a separate book. The issues arise in the historical advantages and disadvantages that other countries have experienced in nationalized or a socialized medicine. The obvious benefit would be that all patients would be covered and no one would be without care when they need it. Unfortunately, the converse side is that these historical models—implemented in Canada, Australia, the United Kingdom, and many European nations—can also be very frustrating when addressing the quickness of care in noncritical cases and the early diagnosis and treatment of some illnesses. In some of these countries, patients with noncritical disorders—rural patients in particular—wait months and in some cases even longer for surgical and/or sometimes diagnostic treatments. The lack of choices for the patient and the inability of the patient to control his or her own healthcare decisions in some cases can lead to the patient being unable to receive care in time to save his or her life.

On the other side, here in the United States, where fewer and fewer individuals are privileged to have jobs that provide any health insurance, the increasing number of citizens who have lost medical insurance for their families are even more deprived than those qualifying to receive socialized medicine. Although patients covered under socialized medical plans may not receive treatment in a timely fashion, individuals without healthcare insurance may not receive any treatment at all. They are simply denied because of inability to pay. This is seen with increasing frequency as the American "middle class" becomes a shrinking economic presence.

Socialized medicine would also raise taxes in a country where increasingly more jobs have gone overseas. In a nation experiencing such great economic shifts, there are no clear-cut solutions. The controversy has many sides. Fortunately, new and improved models of healthcare are being tested overseas. As we watch and look forward to the development of needed changes in our healthcare system, the eventual approach will need to be decided on the basis of virtuous intentions and not shaded by conflicts of interest politically or financially.

Conclusion

Bioethical issues abound in our current society of recent advances in medicine. As we learn increasingly more about genetics and advances in procedures, treatments, and disease prevention, the ethical issues will expand as well. Keeping in mind the basic principles of ethics and ethical decision making, the future can hold astounding cures and treatments for patients who would have died a decade or two ago. Who would have guessed 15 years ago that it would be possible for a patient to live with an artificial heart? We have seen medicine evolve from application of leeches and the use of crude methods of surgical procedures, to the discovery of penicillin and other medications, to the advancement of treatments for heart disease, cancer, kidney failure, and organ transplants. The future will hold even more amazing discoveries and life-prolonging and life-enhancing methods. Of course, the medical and bioethical issues will follow right along with them, so keeping in mind basic ethical principles will become even more important to medical professionals as we journey forward.

Chapter Review Questions

1. What is a double-blind test?
   A. All participants receive the same drug.
   B. All participants have to sign waivers.
   C. No participants are paid for participation.
   D. None of the participants or evaluators know who is receiving the real drug or the placebo.

2. In vitro fertilization involves
   A. use of a surrogate.
   B. harvesting ova to mix with sperm and grow outside the uterus.
   C. artificial insemination.
   D. implantation of embryonic stem cells.

3. Advance directives include
   A. DNR.
   B. patient's wishes for artificial intervention to sustain life.
   C. patient's wishes for healthcare proxy.
   D. All the above

4. What do we mean by a nontherapeutic research group?
   A. Participants do not benefit from research done.
   B. Participants benefit from research done.
   C. No actual participants are used.
   D. Research focuses only on equipment.

5. Palliative means
   A. to aid in death.
   B. to add or extend time to life.
   C. to ease.
   D. to end.

Self-Reflection Questions

1. In your opinion, what ethical issues surrounding medical research trials seem most controversial?
2. What criteria should be in place to prevent a fraudulent medical research study from being published and adapted?
3. What is the worst complicating impact that could occur in a surrogate motherhood case?
4. Should a patient who is suicidal be allowed to refuse treatments to artificially sustain life (e.g., inserting a feeding tube)?

Internet Activities

1. What are the ethical issues surrounding physician-assisted suicides using either passive or active euthanasia?
2. Look up a case called *The Radiation Experiment* and discuss it with others in your class.
3. Find a medical definition of "vegetative state." Then search the Internet for blogs or personal Web pages in which the host discusses a personal experience with a family member or friend who they understood to be in a "vegetative state." On the basis of your findings, what challenges do you imagine facing in helping family members to truly understand what is meant by this term?

Bibliography

Bialik C: The unhealthy accounting of uninsured Americans, *The Wall Street Journal*, June 24, 2009, A12. Found at http://online.wsj.com/article/SB124579852347944191.html. Accessed October 1, 2009.

BMJ 342:c7452, 2011. Found at www.bmj.com/content/342/bmj.c7452.

Hodgson H: A statement by The Royal Free and University College Medical School and The Royal Free Hampstead NHS Trust, *Lancet* 363:824, 2004. Found at http://download.thelancet.com/flatcontentassets/pdfs/S0140673610601754.pdf.

National Institutes of Health (NIH), U.S. Department of Health and Human Services (DHHS): *Research ethics and stem cells*, 2012. Found at http://stemcells.nih.gov/info/pages/ethics.aspx.

New York Times: Opinion: "Justice for all in the baby M case," *New York Times*, February 4, 1988. Found online at www.nytimes.com/1988/02/04/opinion/justice-for-all-in-the-baby-m-case.html.

Publishers of *The Lancet: Retraction—ileal-lymphoid-nodular hyperplasia, non-specific colitis, and pervasive developmental disorder in children*, published online February 2, 2010. DOI: 10.1016/S0140-6736(10)60175-4.

Wakefield AJ, Murch SH, Anthony A et al: Ileal-lymphoid-nodular hyperplasia, non-specific colitis, and pervasive developmental disorder in children, *Lancet* 351:637-641, 1998. Found at http://download.thelancet.com/flatcontentassets/pdfs/S0140673610601754.pdf.

Additional Resources

www.cnn.com/2011/HEALTH/01/06/autism.vaccines/index.html
www.briandeer.com/mmr/lancet-paper.htm
www.cdc.gov/tuskegee/timeline.htm
www.msu.edu/course/hm/546/tuskegee.htm
www.nytimes.com/.../04/opinion/justice-for-all-in-the-baby-m-case.html
www.thevanishingoath.com/
www.pbs.org/independentlens/stemcell/bioethics.html

Chapter 4

Workplace Issues

Jeanne McTeigue

KEY TERMS

Americans with Disabilities Act of 1990 (ADA) Laws enacted in 1990 to protect citizens with disabilities from discrimination.

Chief complaint (CC) The main reason that the patient is being seen by a provider.

Clearinghouse An entity that processes electronic transactions into HIPAA-standardized transactions for billing submission. May also provide billing edits for providers for claims submissions.

Contracts An agreement voluntarily joined by two parties. These can be verbal or written and can be expressed or implied.

Discrimination Treatment of a person or thing, either in opposition of or in favor of, based on bias or prejudice.

Due process Procedures or actions followed to safeguard individual rights. In the workplace, the process to safeguard an employee if he or she feels his or her rights are in jeopardy.

Electronic health record or electronic medical record (EHR/EMR) Software systems that contain the medical records of individuals electronically under HIPAA standards for privacy and security.

Employment-at-will The employment contract that allows an employer to fire or discharge an employee without showing just cause for the termination.

Equal Employment Opportunity Act of 1972 Act that prohibits employment discrimination on the basis of race, color, national origin, sex, religion, age, disability, political beliefs, and marital or familial status.

Occupational Safety and Health Act of 1970 Act that defines and enforces safety regulations for the health and protection of employees in the workplace.

Occupational Safety and Health Administration (OSHA) Federal agency within the Department of Labor that designs, regulates, and monitors standards for employee safety.

Protected health information (PHI) Information about any individual that is identifiable and private about that individual (e.g., Social Security number, date of birth). Public information, such as name and address, is not considered PHI.

Qui tam (whistleblower) In Latin meaning "who as well"; this is the term used for a private citizen who exposes and sues a company or organization that is violating a law and/or breaching a contract with the government. In such cases, the whistleblower may be entitled to a percentage amount or settlement reward for the disclosure of the illegal action.

Sexual harassment Use of power or intimidation over an individual for sexual favors; unwanted or unwelcomed sexual advances and actions or behaviors with sexual implications or innuendoes leading another individual to feel uncomfortable or offended.

SOAP Documentation acronym standing for Subjective, Objective, Assessment, and Plan.

Wrongful discharge A situation when an employee alleges cause that the employment contract or agreement was terminated unjustly or unfairly and therefore the employment contract was breached. The termination of an employee without just cause, without following proper procedures or without due process.

CHAPTER OBJECTIVES

1. List at least two professional qualities necessary for healthcare employment.
2. Delineate key factors in appropriate hiring and firing regulations.
3. Define and categorize types of workplace discrimination.
4. Explain sexual harassment and describe appropriate corporate responses to sexual harassment in the workplace.
5. Describe *qui tam* and its role in healthcare.
6. Outline OSHA and CLIA regulations for workplace safety.
7. Describe two ways to organize key contents in a medical record.
8. Detail issues of ownership related to medical records.
9. Discuss privacy and HIPAA regulations as they pertain to medical records.
10. Name some key guidelines for retention and maintenance of medical records.

Introduction

When an employer has well-defined policies and procedures presented in an employment package for their new hires, the expectations are clearly understood and easily enforced. They protect both the employer and the employee: they may protect the employer from possible *respondeat superior* litigation in the event of an employee working outside the defined job description or in the medical field outside the scope of practice, and they protect both employer and employee through every phase, from hiring through firing.

In addition, employers have an obligation to their employees to provide a safe, unimpeded work environment. In turn, it is the duty of the employees to uphold the standards established by the employer and to perform their duties as defined by their job description with efficiency and productiveness.

Professionalism

No matter how skilled or well-trained an individual may be, a lack of professionalism and "soft skills" may prevent a person from being interviewed or offered employment opportunities. A lack of social skills may even cause a highly qualified professional to lose any job in a short amount of time, even if they do get hired initially.

High levels of professionalism are essential in the medical field. Employers need employees who can conduct themselves professionally and appropriately in all circumstances. Some of these professional qualities include being dependable, hard-working, and able to work well with others and to work without any distractions from personal problems. Anyone can be trained to take a blood pressure reading or measure other vital signs, for example, but it is not always as easy to train an employee to handle a patient with respect and empathy, to be dependable and reliable, or to get along with coworkers.

The truly professional employee leaves personal problems out of the work environment and maintains a high level of integrity. A true professional does not react to situations with emotion but with thoughtful assessment and appropriate response. Professionalism encompasses all the behaviors of an individual, also including the individual's language and appearance. Of course, in an ideal world, all healthcare workers/providers would possess the highest level of professionalism, but even in this less than ideal world, it is essential that we strive for the highest level of integrity and professionalism at all times. All healthcare agencies or facilities proclaim a patient's right declaration or mission statement demanding that patients be treated with dignity and respect. Such respect is essential to ensure the efficient and effective care for all our patients.

What If?

A coworker has been coming into work repeatedly late and seems very preoccupied with issues she is having outside of work. Her performance has been unusually poor and she is acting in a rude and unacceptable way towards the patients; yesterday she told you that she had just been given a verbal warning. Now, this morning, she is late again and has called to ask you to cover for her until she can report to work.

1. How do you handle the continued behavior that you are witnessing?

Hiring and Firing

Policies and procedures outlined in an employee handbook should include specific steps in the process for both hiring and job termination for the organization. Hiring policies should address interviewing and orienting new employees, starting with employment application requirements and any required documentation needed (e.g., licenses) for employment. Company policy regarding advancement and hiring from within the organization should also be addressed in the handbook.

Upon being hired, it is preferable that an individual receives a written contract indicating the job description, salary offered, and start date of the position. However, some agencies or positions are still based on verbal or implied contracts, which are a bit riskier for both sides. Another variation is the practice of hiring an employee "at will." An employment-at-will is designed so that either party may discontinue the employment agreement at any time. These may be found and even presented as a contract, in the example of a per diem or temporary employee. For at-will employees, there is no need to follow protocols for termination; instead, the agreement itself dictates that this type of employee may be discharged without cause. Reasons for firing or terminating a regular employee, however, should be explicitly described in the policies and procedures. This is essential for all employees to feel assured that they will be treated fairly and that due process will be followed.

So what kinds of steps should be included when outlining termination policy? To begin, a manual or policy should clearly define possible consequences of the violation of any company policy. Many policies include a three-step model for corrective action with employees. Most have an initial verbal warning followed by a written warning, and then a third offense would be cause for termination. All employers and/or managers should document accurately any formal action taken with an employee. Some employers identify offenses that would be "grounds for immediate dismissal," and these include extreme offenses such as Health Insurance Portability and Accountability Act (HIPAA) violations or embezzlement. Again, the importance of clear and defined expectations and the clear-cut and defined measures that would be taken if these expectations are violated is essential for any employer, but especially in the medical field where patients' lives are at stake. Errors in judgment or acts of impulsiveness and/or arrogance can lead to severe consequences in the treatment and care of patients.

Discrimination

Laws and regulations concerning the hiring of new employees often center on preventing discrimination. These include specific regulations for interviewing questions and employment application questions. The following is a list of questions that cannot be asked during a job interview.

Illegal Interview Questions

- **Age:** You may ask if a person is between 17 and 70 years old but not specifically ask the person's age.
- **Religion:** You may not ask the candidate's religious background.
- **Race or color:** You may not ask a candidate's race, color, nationality, or heritage.
- **Children:** It is illegal to ask whether the candidate has children or daycare issues.
- **Height and weight:** It is illegal to ask questions about a candidate's height or weight, although equipment restrictions can be shared and explained.
- **Disabilities:** It is illegal to ask whether the candidate has a disability or disease, but it is legal to ask if the candidate has any physical impairment that would prevent him or her from performing the position for which he or she has applied.
- **Arrest records:** A person may have been arrested but not convicted of a crime, so it is illegal to ask whether they have ever been arrested. It is permissible to ask whether someone has been convicted of a felony.
- **Maiden name:** This should only be requested if there is a need to clarify a difference in name upon review of licenses or educational verifications; otherwise, it is an illegal question.

Other areas that are legal, but advisable, to question only as related to the position for application include the following: languages spoken, birthplace, marital status, citizenship, organizations or affiliations, or military experience.

In other words, a good rule of thumb is to avoid raising questions about anything that does not directly pertain to the ability of the individual to perform the duties of the position for which he or she is applying; only ask questions that directly relate to the position at hand.

Antidiscrimination Legislation

The Civil Rights Act of 1964 and the Equal Employment Opportunity Act of 1972 were two landmark laws that required that all persons must be treated equally and be given the same opportunities for employment and advancement in the workforce in all areas. Categories of discrimination in employment have been committed historically in the areas of race, religion, color, age, gender, family situation, nationality, and sexual orientation. These two laws have gone far in protecting against these discriminations in both hiring practices and **wrongful discharge**.

Another area of discrimination was found to occur against disabled Americans, thus prompting the enactment of the **Americans with Disabilities Act (ADA) of 1990** and its predecessor, the Rehabilitation Act of 1973. Under these laws, if a candidate applies for enrollment in an educational facility or an employment opportunity, the Americans with Disabilities Act provides that the candidate can expect "reasonable" accommodations if necessary and should not be discriminated against in the pursuit of employment, education, or access to public places because of the disability. The following is an example of the way this Act may be implemented. Suppose an employee is hired and is confined to a wheelchair. He or she may file a Form 504, requesting the accommodation of a work station with wheelchair accessibility. The phrase "reasonable accommodations" refers to necessary and appropriate changes to any system or structure that would make the environment equal and fair. The full listing of and complete guidelines for reasonable accommodations can be found on the Equal Employment Opportunity Commission (EEOC) website found at the following link: www.eeoc.gov/policy/docs/accommodation.html.

In the medical field we must be ready to accommodate and show sensitivity to individuals who may have cultural or religious beliefs with which we may not agree. Autonomy would dictate that our patients have the right to make choices based on their beliefs, and we must respect those rights. The only exception occurs when a minor child's life is in danger and the hospital or healthcare provider may deem it necessary to intercede on behalf of the minor child's life, safety, or health.

Sexual Harassment

Sexual harassment is the intimidation of another or unwanted advances or sexual comments that cause another person to feel uncomfortable (Figure 4-1). Sexual harassment is an offense of discrimination according to the Civil Rights Amendment of 1964. Unwanted sexual advances or requests for sexual favors, as well as other actions or conversations of a sexual nature, can mean criminal charges brought against the offender. For the employee, it could be grounds for immediate dismissal or, at the least, corrective action, depending on the offense. Guidelines on sexual harassment are clear and can be reviewed at www.eeoc.gov/eeoc/publications/fs-sex.cfm. Per the EEOC guidelines, the victim should make it clear to the harasser that the actions are unwanted and unacceptable. If the action does not stop immediately, the victim should then inform management and follow internal complaint policies. The EEOC will perform investigations in these matters and the complaining individual does not have to be the person who was harassed but can also be anyone who was affected by the incident. The offender can be a male or a female and the offense can be from either an opposite or a same-sex individual.

Most employers have policies and procedures in place to follow when such incidents occur. These procedures include steps for reporting, following up, and discontinuing any harassment conduct, as well as provisions for charging or terminating an offender.

Qui Tam

The Latin phrase *qui tam* means "who as well" and is the term used for a private citizen who exposes and sues a company or organization that is violating the law and/or

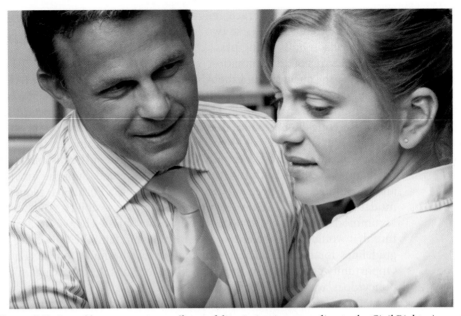

Figure 4-1 Sexual harassment is an offense of discrimination according to the Civil Rights Amendment of 1964.

Discussion

Several coworkers are in the lunch room on their lunch break. Sam and his friend George are having a rather loud conversation about the party they attended over the past weekend. George relates a joke that he heard at the party and it is a very sexually oriented joke with several words that offend Sally (who overhears the conversation). Sally is upset and makes a complaint to them about the nature of the conversation that they are having and how it is offensive to her. George and Sam tell her that she is overreacting and dismiss her complaint.

1. Is this considered sexual harassment?
2. Can any actions be taken to follow up on this incident?
3. Is Sally just overreacting to the situation?

breaching the contract with the government. In such cases, the "whistleblower" may be entitled to a percentage amount or settlement reward for the uncovering of the illegal action.

"Whistleblowers" is a common term attached to private individuals who file lawsuits against agencies or companies that are in violation of government laws or regulations. In cases of violations of workplace laws, an individual can file their information with the appropriate authorities. In *qui tam* cases, the individual may be entitled to reimbursement or a reward for the disclosure of the offender. For example, a violation may have specific fines and penalties attached, and a whistleblower may gain a percentage financially if the case is tried by the government and the *qui tam* individual is named as the complaining party.

Most healthcare cases that are *qui tam* cases have been fraud and abuse related, but any violation of government regulations or laws can be considered *qui tam*.

What If?

A new employee is working in the billing and accounting department of a group practice of physicians. The new employee has the responsibility of opening the insurance checks from the mail and posting the payments into the system. The checks are then totalled and deposited in the company bank account. One of the physicians has approached the new employee on a few occasions and has taken the checks from her to "handle" them himself. This makes the employee feel uncomfortable because it seems slightly peculiar that this one physician is taking the checks but not the other monies that should be deposited with them.

1. What should the new employee do?

Safety in the Workplace

The employer is responsible to ensure that all areas of the workplace are safe for both employees and patients. All physical hazard spaces, medical waste, and medical biohazards (such as used sharps) must be handled following specific guidelines initiated by the Occupational Safety and Health Act of 1970. The Occupational Safety and Health Administration (OSHA) has been established for all kinds of businesses and safeguards employees from potential risks for illness or injury. Regulations under OSHA encompass everything from ergonomic work stations to lumbar support braces for heavy lifting, protective gloves, eye-wash stations, and goggles and gowns, establishing standards for all employees who are at risk for injury or infection (Figure 4-2). Especially as it pertains to healthcare, OSHA requires personal protection equipment (PPE) that is designed to protect healthcare workers from exposure to contagious

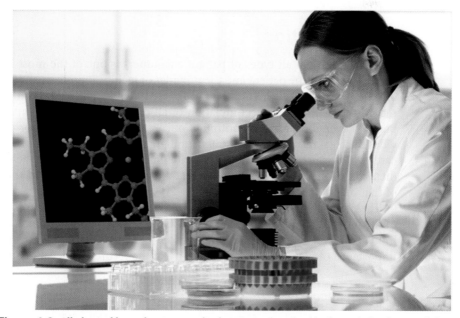

Figure 4-2 All physical hazard spaces, medical waste, and medical biohazards (such as used sharps) must be handled following specific guidelines initiated by OSHA.

illnesses as well as injuries from equipment or instruments that can be sharp or dangerous. OSHA has been the driving force for many of the safeguards that we see now, such as "wet floor" signs. OSHA also mandates that healthcare workers who are at risk of exposure should be immunized for various diseases, such as hepatitis B. Other guidelines include the elimination of contaminated materials and disposal of sharps and other biohazard materials. Through OSHA, Materials Substance Data Sheets (MSDSs) were developed so that all workplaces would have a guide for the steps to take in cases of exposure. The sheets include all substances, ranging from Wite-Out correction fluid to formaldehyde. Finally, OSHA mandates annual in-service training for those staff regularly exposed to blood-borne pathogens and infectious diseases, and most healthcare facilities must include mandatory fire safety and first aid/cardiopulmonary resuscitation (CPR) training as well.

All employees should follow the guidelines for their particular area from the OSHA mandates, and some facilities will even encourage steps beyond the minimum OSHA requirements to ensure the health and well-being of their employees.

CLIA, the Clinical Laboratory Improvement Act of 1988, regulates all laboratory facilities for safety and handling of specimens. All laboratories are given a CLIA number and are required to maintain certain standards of operation.

What If?

Sandra is a nurse in the physician's office and she has just assisted the physician with a suturing procedure. As she is cleaning up afterwards, she is cut by the suture needle and it penetrates her glove.

1. What procedures should be followed?
2. Is the employer responsible even though Sandra made the mistake?
3. How does this incident affect the patient whose blood is on the suture needle?
4. Can the patient be forced to have HIV testing?

Documentation

Documentation of all types of patient encounters is one of the most important parts of healthcare for the patient and the provider or facility. It protects all parties by recording the details of each encounter and the treatment performed. For the patient it is a record that will give an accumulation of all diagnoses and treatments that affect the patient's overall health and continuity of care. For the facility and/or provider, it provides the legal record of all treatment and physical findings. The golden rule of healthcare is "if it is not documented, it did not happen." Providers must be diligent in their dictation of the events of all encounters and must understand that the thoroughness of that record is essential.

The completeness, timeliness, and accuracy of the medical records are paramount to the protection of the patient and provider and cannot be considered flippantly. Any individual who is documenting data into the medical record needs to appreciate the importance of maintaining the credibility of the record as a legal document.

Medical Record

Depending on the place of service, the medical record can differ in how it is organized, what it contains, and who is responsible for maintaining the records. For instance, in the hospital setting, generally, the patient is assigned a medical record number, which always stays the same; however, each *encounter* that same patient has with the hospital is assigned an account number. In other words, if the patient, for example, a 16-year-old male, has his tonsils removed and then 6 months later has a broken ankle set in the emergency department, that patient will always have the same medical record number at that hospital. However, the tonsillectomy and the ankle surgery will each be assigned separate, new account numbers under that medical record number. This makes both billing and coding—as well as medical follow-up—easier in tracking the two separate encounters.

Charting varies too. For example, when a patient is seen as an outpatient, the documentation is simple and may only consist of a few items (e.g., drawing blood for analysis), but if that same patient is admitted as an inpatient or is having surgery performed, then a full chart is compiled and the reports and documentation for those encounters will be much more involved. In an inpatient chart, several individuals are responsible for the documentation of the hospital stay, such as nurses, anesthesiologists, and technicians, as well as the physicians who are managing the patient and the possible consulting physicians who may see the patient.

In the office setting, the documentation of the patient is generally one chart per patient and contains all the encounters for that patient in that single record. Most outpatient charts are organized chronologically with the most recent information on top. Some may vary with organization of the chart by problem or diagnosis, known as the "problem-oriented medical record" (POMR) format, but the majority of outpatient records store information in a chronological format.

Elements of the Medical Record

The main elements of the medical record may vary depending on the place of service, but the general categories seen in virtually all medical records tend to include the following:

Demographic—The patient's identifying information, such as name, address, Social
   Security number, date of birth, and insurance information.
Progress notes—Office or encounter notes by the staff and providers indicating the
   findings of exams, review of body systems (ROS), and history from the patient.
   These may also include the patient's record of medications and notes from phone
   calls with the patient as well as recommendations and referrals. The information
   may be office notes documented in the SOAP format or reports documented in the
   CHEDDAR format (see the following boxes describing these formats).
Labs and testing—Lab reports of blood work, urinalysis, minor biopsies, tuberculosis
   (TB) tests, or any reports from other testing or consults done for the patient.

SOAP and CHEDDAR Formats

Many forms used to document general examination and treatment visits with patients use the acronym SOAP to organize patient progress notes. The initials SOAP may appear in the margins of the form or may be in title sections on the electronic health record (electronic medical record, EHR/EMR). These stand for the following elements of documentation:

Another common format is used to provide a more detailed report or record; it uses the acronym CHEDDAR to guide the documentation's organization. As you can see in the box that follows, the elements are the same as those in SOAP notes, but they are more detailed and expanded.

Many medical records, depending on the type and the manner in which they are organized, may detail these formats into many subsections but the basic content of the information is similar.

SOAP

S–Subjective: History given by patient, including **chief complaint (CC)**;
history of present illness (HPI); and any past, family, and social history taken
(PFSH)
O–Objective: Examination findings and any test results reviewed
A–Assessment: Diagnosis and summation of the provider's impressions
P–Plan: Treatment and/or follow-up plans for the patient, including any
medications or tests ordered

CHEDDAR

C–Chief complaint (CC)
H–History of present illness (HPI)
E–Examination
D–Details
D–Drugs and dosages
A–Assessment
R–Return to office

Reasons for Documentation

No matter what setting medical records are documented, the medical record serves
several purposes:

Legal: First and foremost, it is a legal document and can be subpoenaed for legal
purposes, such as a criminal act or any lawsuit.
Fraud: The record also serves as a record of proof for the providers against fraud from
insurance companies by validating that what was billed was actually performed.
Continuity of care: It can be vital to a patient's health that a medical record can be
shared with other providers to show the flow of the care given. This is also important
for the portability of the records should the patient relocate.
Malpractice: A medical record is the main source for defense in any malpractice suit
that may arise, protecting the provider by verifying the events of each encounter
with the patient.

For all these reasons, documentation in the medical record must always be done
legibly, effectively, and accurately. It is vital that providers and staff realize the serious-
ness of their impact on patients' future treatment and progress by ensuring that the
correct information is documented and the integrity of the records is preserved.

Correction and Amendments to the Medical Record

Clearly, we are human, and errors in the medical record can occur. If an error occurs
in a written record, the ONLY acceptable way to correct that mistake is to (1) draw a
single line through the error, (2) write the corrected entry above it, and (3) initial and
date the correction.

In dictated or typed notes, if a provider has forgotten to add something, it is acceptable for the provider to dictate an addendum to that note. Every note or change dictated
must be (1) initialed and dated by the transcriptionist who types it, and then (2)
approved by the provider by adding his or her initials and date. This final initially and

dating by the provider is the official indication that the provider has read the final, typed document and approved its accuracy. If there are errors in the dictation, the provider should not sign-off on it until the copy is corrected. It is the provider's responsibility to review these documents carefully for the completeness and accuracy of the typed document.

Ownership

Many patients have trouble understanding that they do not "own" their medical records. Although a medical record is "about" a patient, it does not belong to that individual. Instead, it is the provider's or physician's instrument for recording or documenting all treatment and assessments of the patient; it is a record of their work with that patient. In fact, all testing and examinations have reviews documented by the physicians who provided that care, and it is documented mainly not only to ensure continuity of care but also to provide protection and a legal record. It is the physician's tool for helping to ensure continuity of care for the patient as well. Lack of any documentation by the provider can be viewed as negligence to the patient and in some states can be reason for revocation of the provider's license.

Although the medical record is clearly the provider's property, each patient does have the right to copies of those records. Records can be copied and transferred to other physicians under the patient's consent, but the originals of those records belong to the provider or facility.

Privacy and Release of Information

Release of information from the provider, on behalf of the patient, is only done with a signed written release from the patient. This ensures that the identifying and private information in the medical record is protected from public knowledge. HIPAA ensures that a patient's personal, identifying health records should be protected by law; violations can result in fines and penalties up to $10,000 and possible imprisonment.

There are only a few instances in which there is no requirement for a release or authorization from the patient for release of information. These situations include the following:

1. Criminal acts (e.g., crucial evidence for abuse cases, stabbings, gunshot wounds, rapes)
2. Legally ordered (e.g., court orders or subpoena of records, regardless of whether for criminal cases)
3. Communicable diseases (the Centers for Disease Control and Prevention or local health departments can require release of information in case of the possibility of diseases that potentially could cause pandemic or sexually transmitted diseases, such as human immunodeficiency virus [HIV], syphilis, bubonic plague, severe acute respiratory syndrome [SARS], whooping cough, or tuberculosis)
4. Mandated (e.g., examinations ordered by employers' insurance companies for workers' compensation cases, court orders)

Health Insurance Portability and Accountability Act of 1996 (HIPAA)

The Health Insurance Portability and Accountability Act of 1996 (HIPAA) was designed to protect the privacy of sensitive patient information and combat fraud in the health-care industry, simplify administration of health insurance, and promote the use of medical savings plans for employees. The law itself has five titles within it that cover portability, administrative simplification, medical savings and tax deductions, group health plan provisions, and revenue offset provisions. Title II focuses on Administrative Simplification and the Privacy Rule, which we will examine next.

The Privacy Rule

As more and more patient records become electronically stored, new complications arise that were not as pertinent with paper records. The medical community and members of Congress realized that streamlining the processing of healthcare information could place the patient's private information at risk. In response to this, the Department of Health and Human Services (HHS) was assigned the task of safeguarding patients' **protected health information (PHI)**, resulting in the establishment in 2001 of the Privacy Rule. To ensure the electronic safety of the widespread sharing of patient information, the HHS mandated in this ruling that all "covered entities" submitting electronic information would have to be in compliance with the electronic code set, privacy, and security of PHI by April 14, 2003. This means implementing standardization of guidelines for electronic language or code sets as well as the security of physical and electronic devices. The standards aim specifically at protecting health information electronically submitted from providers to **clearinghouses** and then to the individual carriers. In addition, both carriers and providers were mandated to update language and software into compliance with the universal format called 837 or ANSI format (computer language) by April 2003. In other words, the new law required all covered entities or business associates in the healthcare field to convert all electronic transmission to this universal format, and to send any form of electronic transmission of files or patient information under the secure code sets designated by OCR and HHS. Now, at the time of this writing, new updates are being added to cover the incoming ICD-10 diagnostic codes that will be mandated for use in October of 2014.

Other strategies that entities and related staff commit to under HIPAA agreements include protecting the safety of the physical chart and identifying physical information through individual password protection, screen shut-down for monitors left idle, and other electronic code set criteria.

Finally, now patients are routinely asked to sign-off on paperwork, acknowledging that they have read and comply with the HIPAA policy notification with any healthcare provider or facility from which they seek care. It has also become standard for releases to be signed as needed for transmission of information to insurance carriers, as well as signing releases that indicate whether or not a phone message may be left on the patient's home phone. All these help to safeguard the patient's rights to privacy.

What If?

A medical assistant is at the local store and notices a patient who had been in the office that morning. The patient is with her husband, and the medical assistant greets the patient and congratulates her on the "good news." The patient is upset, and the medical assistant realizes not only that the patient had not yet informed her husband of the pregnancy but also that the husband had previously undergone a vasectomy and was not the father.
1. What could happen to the medical assistant for this incident?
2. Would this be considered a mistake rather than an actual violation of HIPAA?
3. Would the employer be responsible for the medical assistant's violation?

National Provider Identifier (NPI)

Other than the Privacy Rule, the most common title of the HIPAA law that affects all healthcare providers, staff, and facilities is Title II—Administrative Simplification. The idea behind this part of HIPAA was to streamline the flow of information and to make a uniform system that would be used universally by providers and insurance companies. Previously, as an example, each individual insurance company would have a credentialing process and paperwork that the individual providers would have to submit to become participating providers for that insurance company; sometimes individual providers would need to complete separate credentialing packets for different plans within the insurance companies. This process could not be duplicated from one carrier to another and there was no central information center that could be accessed by all carriers.

The HIPAA laws provided for the NPI or National Provider Identifier, whereby each provider files credentials with the national database (Centers for Medicare and Medicaid Services), and each provider is issued one NPI to be used for all the different area insurance carriers with which the provider works. This provides an effective way of streamlining the administrative areas of healthcare by eliminating the need for several different provider identification numbers. A single identification number is transmitted electronically instead of needing different programming for each electronic form sent to each specific carrier.

As we move forward in the electronic age of medicine, we are now able to transmit and make portable much of the patient's records. The ability to send a magnetic resonance imaging (MRI) scan to an orthopedic surgeon and the capacity to forward a prescription refill or order to the pharmacy are just a couple of the newly developed improvements in the healthcare of individuals attributable to the advancements in electronic media.

Whether via social networking or emails, there has to be very careful deliberation about the information that can be added to the Internet. Many practices and facilities now have their own websites. The electronic use of software to research drug interactions and resource information for patients while they are in the office and also the ability to submit referrals and requests for appointments online have the potential to advance our ability to serve our patients better. This is a vital resource for medicine in the future but we must be mindful that such vast use and access is a vulnerable place for HIPAA violations. The HIPAA compliance of these compatible programs needs to be secure and managed carefully to protect the safety and security of the information that is being transmitted.

> **?** **What If?**
> A physician in the emergency department is trying to ask another physician (i.e., a friend) about a drug interaction that he suspects in his patient. He messages his friend on a social networking site to ask the question. Would this be a HIPAA violation?

Retention and Maintenance of Medical Records

Regulations on storing and maintaining records vary among each state regarding how long they must be saved. The majority of records are stored approximately 10 years from the final entry of the record. Because of today's litigious environment, however, most providers do not destroy any medical records. Even if a patient is deceased, the providers may microfiche or store inactive files in a secure storage facility, but they usually do not destroy the documentation. With the upcoming transition to electronic health records, storage will be easier to maintain for providers because the written documents can be scanned into the medical electronic record and, once confirmed, may be shredded or filed in long-term storage. Any vital statistics on a patient must be kept permanently, such as birth or death records, immunization records, and chemotherapy treatment records.

Most providers will not, for their own protection, destroy a record, but if one is lost or misplaced, it can be damaging to both patient and provider. Most cases of litigation would tend to not look at a lost record as an accident but as a deliberate attempt to hide a file from discovery. If electronic records are not practical in some situations, it can be wise to take other precautions, which could include the following: a log or sign-out for medical records removed from the files; a system of filing with color coding to enable visual clues to charts that are misfiled; and the designation of a specific person to both manage and verify records for accuracy, regularly auditing files for their completeness, and working continually to track any missing files.

Conclusion

In all workplace environments there should be an assigned "chain of command" to follow any complaints within the work environment. A hostile or uncomfortable workplace is difficult, at best, to handle, but proper procedures and policies should help to defend the employee and protect the employer in all situations that might arise. In the medical profession this should be especially true and indeed the highest standards of professionalism and ethical behavior are expected and should be upheld.

The medical record and documentation of medical care is a legal catalog of the patient's individual encounters and treatments that provides the proof and legal justifications for the providers and also allows portability of records for the patients. In the advancement of electronic records now and in the future, the patient's continuity of care and ability to access healthcare will become more streamlined and effective. It is important as we move forward to always bear in mind that the safeguard of the information we have on patients and the security and integrity of the information should be of the utmost importance.

Chapter Review Questions

1. What organization oversees the enforcement of equal rights and fights discrimination?
   A. CMS
   B. OSHA
   C. EEOC
   D. HIPAA

2. What is another name for whistleblower?
   A. *Qui tam*
   B. *Respondeat superior*
   C. OSHA
   D. Subpoena *duces tecum*

3. What is the definition of PHI?
   A. Possible health information
   B. Protected health information
   C. Protected health insurance
   D. Possible health insurance

4. What is a component of S in SOAP?
   A. Exam
   B. History
   C. Test results
   D. All of the above

5. Where would you find the medication information for the patient in CHEDDAR?
   A. C
   B. H
   C. D
   D. R

Self-Reflection Questions

1. What discriminations have you felt victim of in the past? What would you do if you were a witness to another employee being subjected to discrimination?
2. What OSHA guidelines directly affect you in the workplace?
3. Is there an area of your own profession that should be more closely monitored for HIPAA compliance? How well does your current facility seem to recognize the full impact and vital importance of documentation?

Internet Activities

1. Look up *qui tam* under the guidelines of Medicare at the website www.cms.gov.
2. Using the website www.eeoc.gov/eeoc/publications/fs-sex.cfm find the EEOC guidelines regarding sexual harassment and investigate the different forms.
3. Using the following website, determine the types of entities covered by CMS guidelines: http://www.cms.gov/Regulations-and-Guidance/HIPAA-Administrative-Simplification/HIPAAGenInfo/AreYouaCoveredEntity.html.

Additional Resources

http://civilrights.findlaw.com/discrimination/
   the-americans-with-disabilities-act-overview

http://findlaw.com/discrimination

http://uslegal.com

http://eeoc.gov

http://www.cms.gov

http://ada.gov

http://www.eeoc.gov/eeoc/publications/fs-sex.cfm

http://www.hhs.gov/ocr/privacy/hipaa/understanding/index.html

www.cms.gov

www.ama-assn.org

www.ocr.gov

http://www.cms.gov/Regulations-and-Guidance/HIPAA-Administrative-
   Simplification/HIPAAGenInfo/AreYouaCoveredEntity.html

http://www.hhs.gov/ocr/privacy/hipaa/understanding/index.html

http://www.cms.gov/Regulations-and-Guidance/HIPAA-Administrative-
   Simplification/TransactionCodeSetsStands/index.html?redirect=/
   TransactionCodeSetsStands/02_TransactionsandCodeSetsRegulations.
   asp#TopOfPage

Chapter 5

Code and Standards Infractions

Jeanne McTeigue

KEY TERMS

Bias A preference of one thing over another, usually unfairly favoring one over another.

Compliance Adherence to guidelines and regulations set forth by an organization and/or a governing body.

Compliance officer The individual in an organization or practice who is designated to maintain and inspect the adherence of all areas of regulations and guidelines. (In healthcare organizations these officers perform audits and use established checks and balances to prevent fraud and abuse.)

Compliance plan Policies and procedures used to ensure that guidelines and regulations are obeyed, including auditing, monitoring, and protocol for taking action when infractions (whether deliberate or unintentional) are discovered.

Confidentiality Agreement to maintain and respect the privacy of certain information disclosed. In the medical field, applies to patient privacy in particular.

Consumer protection Laws and safeguards to protect consumers from fraudulent, unethical, or illegal practices.

Discrimination Treatment of a person or thing, either unsupportive or supportive, based on bias or prejudice.

Due process Procedures or actions followed to safeguard individual rights. In the workplace, the process to safeguard an employee if he or she feels his or her rights are in jeopardy.

Employment Protection Acts Broad group of acts that govern handling of employees or potential employees. Generally cover the following areas: interviewing, debt collections, interest and charges, equal opportunity employment, disability act, compensation and benefits, antitrust, and antikickback.

Fraud Deliberate, intentional act to mislead for financial gain.

Health Insurance Portability and Accountability Act (HIPAA) Set of laws regulated by the Office for Civil Rights (OCR) that protect and secure the information and privacy of patients. Laws that ensure a patient's rights to privacy and portability of healthcare records transmitted either nonelectronically or electronically.

Medical practice acts Laws defined by each of the states that regulate the licensing and medical laws for that state and define the scope of practice for licensed and unlicensed individuals in the healthcare field.

Occupational Safety and Health Administration (OSHA) Federal agency within the Department of Labor that designs, regulates, and monitors standards for employee safety.

Office for Civil Rights (OCR) Federal office established to uphold the rights of individuals, regarding rights to privacy and standards of care. Enforces HIPAA regulations.

Office of Inspector General (OIG) Independent agency that functions under the Department of Justice to investigate and protect the integrity of the Department of Health and Human Services (HHS) and their recipients, as well as welfare programs.

Protected health information (PHI) Information about any individual that is identifiable and private about that individual (e.g., Social Security number, date of birth). Public information (such as name and address) is not considered PHI.

Sanctions Penalties that can be levied on an individual for violating a policy or rule. (Can also mean permission or agreement in other contexts.)

Sexual harassment Use of power or intimidation over an individual for sexual favors; unwanted or unwelcomed sexual advances and actions or behaviors with sexual implications or innuendoes leading another individual to feel uncomfortable or offended.

Stark laws Laws designed to maintain the integrity of the medical field; include antitrust and antikickback laws to prevent physicians from gaining financially from solicitation of services or monopolization of services.

CHAPTER OBJECTIVES

1. Identify the purpose of disciplinary actions.
2. Explain workplace standards and expectations.
3. List examples of ethical and illegal actions that would warrant disciplinary actions.
4. Outline the basics of a compliance plan.
5. Describe the role of the compliance officer.
6. Describe key types of compliance violations.
7. List federal and state agencies that oversee and resolve matters that require disciplinary action.

Introduction

Employers and official professional bodies such as certification boards, licensing boards, and other agencies of the state and federal government all work together to oversee the medical field to ensure that the rights of patients and the general public are safeguarded. It is the duty of all healthcare professionals to monitor themselves and uphold the ethical standards of the profession. If an individual commits an illegal or unethical act it is the responsibility of the individual's employer or governing body to enforce the sanctions that would be appropriate for the violation that occurred.

Disciplinary Action

Disciplinary actions are consequences that are levied against an individual who has violated either the laws or the ethical standards for that profession. In the medical field violations can range from the unethical treatment of a patient or individual (or negligence of care) to a Health Insurance Portability and Accountability (HIPAA) violation of privacy, fraud, or other illegal actions. In addition to the legal consequences of breaking a law, employers and agencies may also enforce sanctions that extend beyond these legal consequences. Although committing an illegal act may lead to fines and possible imprisonment, professional and workplace sanctions depend on professional codes of conduct (not laws) and may include such corrective actions as termination of employment or loss of license.

Workplace Standards

Every medical or healthcare employer, whether a hospital, agency, or group practice, should have a set of standards defining the expectations of their employees based on their position and expertise. Policies and procedures should be well-defined in the employees' handbook or other employment packets given at the time of hiring and should include a description of the duties or responsibilities of specific positions and the code of ethics or defined standards for that institution (Figure 5-1). As new employees sign-off on such documents, they acknowledge the specified consequences that will result from working outside of the parameters of that job description or violating the code of ethics.

Reasons for Disciplinary Actions

Reasons for disciplinary action vary among states and facilities as well as from one area of expertise to another. State and federal regulations focus on violations in the areas of fraud, substance abuse, illegal acts, operating without a license, acting outside the scope of practice, and malpractice. Illegal and unethical acts can be penalized by law, licensing and/or ethics boards, certification boards, and employers, with consequences varying depending on the severity of the act or lack of action. For example, in the case of a minor infraction, the consequences may just include a corrective action plan (CAP) by an employer or a temporary loss of license or small fine/penalty. In the case of a more serious infraction, the person may incur permanent loss of license and heavy fines and penalties. If a physician, for example, is found to be guilty of substance abuse, the physician may have a loss of license imposed by Medicare or the state licensing board and lose their livelihood.

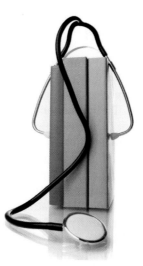

Figure 5-1 Policies and procedures should be well-defined in the employee's handbook or other employment packets and should include a description of duties or responsibilities as well as the code of ethics or defined standards.

Examples of Work-Related Offenses That Could Warrant Disciplinary Action*

Violation of time-off policy or sick-time policy
Violation of dress code policy
Violation of the code of ethics
Violation of duties—either failing to perform job or working outside job description
Violation of the integrity of the institution, such as embezzlement or slander against the institution
Abandonment of responsibility or position
Noncompliance with continuing education or annual in-service requirements
Physical or emotional impairment on the job
Sexual harassment
Assault
Battery
Violation of employment protection acts
Violation of consumer protection acts

*These are only examples and all employers and/or institutions may have several additional areas that are included in their individual policies.

Examples of Work-Related Offenses Specific to Healthcare Professions That Could Warrant Disciplinary Action*

Violation of patient's rights (e.g., HIPAA or confidentiality breach)
Working outside employee's scope of practice
Failure to perform at the accepted standard of care
Fraud/abuse
Abandonment of patient(s)
Falsifying documentation
Lack of documentation
Negligence
Violation of Stark laws

*Again, these are meant to be common examples and are not intended to be "all inclusive."

Compliance Plan

Let us look closer at that compliance plan. Earlier, we mentioned that all employers should have a written policy or new-hire handbook that details expectations and standards for all employees, including, but not be limited to, dress code, code of ethics, and job description. Taking that one step further, it should also detail the measures to be taken in the event of any violation of the company policies.

For example, protected health information (PHI) is information about any individual that is protected by law from being shared or discussed outside proper channels for treatment. This extremely private information includes such crucial data as a person's Social Security number and date of birth. Public information, such as name and address, is not considered PHI. Patients' rights to confidentiality are covered by the Health Insurance Portability and Accountability Act (HIPAA) rules established and regulated by the Office for Civil Rights (OCR).

Suppose, then, that company policy states that a violation of patient confidentiality is grounds for immediate dismissal; then the employee is aware of the consequences for such an action and could not appeal a termination if found guilty of that violation. The employer, in this case, inflicts the consequence of immediate termination, and no further action is necessary from legal or state authorities. Conversely, however, depending on the state and the employee's position, the state may impose fines and court penalties.

HIPAA fines vary but can range up to $10,000 in some states. The point is that the employer's decision to immediately terminate this employee is a matter of company policy documented in a compliance plan.

Due Process

All employees should have a right to due process, which means that an employee has the right to require that all specified procedures outlined in the compliance plan be followed if that employee's employment later is in jeopardy. For example, if an employee is given a verbal warning for a violation and the next step (per the policy) would be a written warning, then the employer cannot just fire the employee arbitrarily without following the steps defined in the policy. These rights are part of a broader umbrella called the Employment Protection Acts—a broad group of acts that govern handling of employees or potential employees.

Most employers have a series of steps that must be taken before an employee can be terminated. For instance, policy may dictate that a first offense incurs a verbal warning; the second offense involves a written or more formal warning; and a third offense will result in termination. The employer must document each step in the employee's file to show that due process was followed and that the policy of the institution was observed.

Failure to provide written policies can be a dangerous position for both employee and employer. With no written policy of expectations, how does an employee know how to meet his or her expectations? Similarly, how does the employer have any power to reprimand or impose sanction on an employee when no policy is in place to explain the expectations? Therefore, a clear policy and procedures manual or employee handbook protects both sides, and in the medical field it also protects the patients.

A compliance plan also helps the organization monitor the employer and the organization itself against possible fraud and abuse of privilege. We will look at these practices in the next section.

What If?

An employee is found to be making errors in documenting a patient's chart and is given a verbal warning for this error. The employee is placed on a corrective action plan and is to receive training on the proper method of documenting a patient's chart. The employee does not comply with the corrective action determined, and the employer fires the employee subsequently.

1. Does the employee have the right to fight the termination of employment based on due process?
2. Does the employer have to offer even more training for the employee?
3. What could the employer or the employee do differently in this case?

Compliance Officer

In a busy work environment, whose responsibility is it to monitor for compliance and violations? To maintain high standards, most healthcare employers designate or hire a specific individual to act as a compliance officer to ensure that these policies and procedures are being obeyed and that any violations are being addressed appropriately. This role may require a separate full-time position in itself, or may be carried out by a supervisor or manager in any given area or department. This individual should be easily identified so that employees can access the officer if they have any questions or concerns regarding compliance and employer policies. A designated compliance officer also serves as a double-check to ensure that all employees are held to these same standards and regulations. It is considered discrimination if a supervisor or employer treats any one individual differently than another.

What If?

A veterinary assistant was originally hired for a full-time position with a handbook that defines "full time" as working 35 hours per week with 1 hour each day for unpaid lunch breaks. After 4 months, a new supervisor is hired in the facility and begins scheduling the full-time employees for 30 hours per week. Unfortunately, this means that the employees will suffer a deduction in pay for 5 hours. When the employees complain, the supervisor says that the facility is cutting back department costs, and she has chosen to reduce costs in this manner.

1. What recourse do the employees have?
2. Is the supervisor justified in her actions?
3. What would be some ideas that would remedy this situation?

Monitoring the Employer or Institution

So, we might ask the following question: If we have all these regulations in place for minding employees, then who is minding the boss? We have seen how a compliance plan helps monitor employee actions, but it is also in place to protect an organization against illegal, fraudulent, or fractious actions of the employer or physician. A number of state and federal agencies help to monitor quality control, safety, ethics, and legal patency of healthcare organizations. For example, the Office of Inspector General (OIG) is an independent agency that functions under the Department of Justice to investigate and protect the integrity of the Department of Health and Human Services (HHS) and their recipients, as well as welfare programs. There are more than 70 OIG offices throughout the United States.

Fraud

We will begin by defining actions that constitute fraud. Fraud is the intentional act to misrepresent facts or mislead in order to gain financially. It is a criminal offense that can lead to providers and billing and coding personnel incurring fines, loss of license, and even imprisonment. Examples of fraud include billing for services not provided, up-coding services for larger reimbursement, or down-coding (under coding) for services provided (Figure 5-2).

Medicare guidelines require proper documentation for services performed: if it is not documented, it did not happen and you cannot bill for it. Many providers are lacking in documentation skills, and as a result, the work performed is not billed. In addition, many providers down-code their services to avoid any indication of fraud, but indeed this too is considered to be fraud, although, unlike falsely billing or coding to increase reimbursement, there are no cases of known prosecution for down-coding.

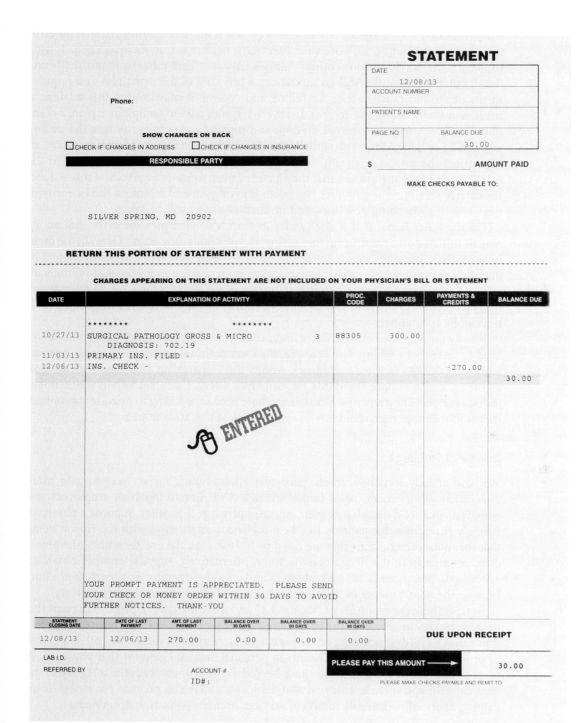

STATEMENT

DATE	
12/08/13	
ACCOUNT NUMBER	
PATIENT'S NAME	
PAGE NO.	BALANCE DUE
	30.00

$ _____ AMOUNT PAID

MAKE CHECKS PAYABLE TO:

Phone:

SHOW CHANGES ON BACK
☐ CHECK IF CHANGES IN ADDRESS   ☐ CHECK IF CHANGES IN INSURANCE
RESPONSIBLE PARTY

SILVER SPRING, MD   20902

RETURN THIS PORTION OF STATEMENT WITH PAYMENT

CHARGES APPEARING ON THIS STATEMENT ARE NOT INCLUDED ON YOUR PHYSICIAN'S BILL OR STATEMENT

DATE	EXPLANATION OF ACTIVITY		PROC. CODE	CHARGES	PAYMENTS & CREDITS	BALANCE DUE
	******** ********					
10/27/13	SURGICAL PATHOLOGY GROSS & MICRO	3	88305	300.00		
	DIAGNOSIS: 702.19					
11/03/13	PRIMARY INS. FILED -					
12/06/13	INS. CHECK -				-270.00	
						30.00

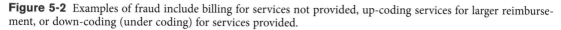 ENTERED

YOUR PROMPT PAYMENT IS APPRECIATED. PLEASE SEND
YOUR CHECK OR MONEY ORDER WITHIN 30 DAYS TO AVOID
FURTHER NOTICES.   THANK-YOU

STATEMENT CLOSING DATE	DATE OF LAST PAYMENT	AMT. OF LAST PAYMENT	BALANCE OVER 30 DAYS	BALANCE OVER 60 DAYS	BALANCE OVER 90 DAYS	DUE UPON RECEIPT
12/08/13	12/06/13	270.00	0.00	0.00	0.00	

LAB I.D.
REFERRED BY   ACCOUNT #
                                     ID#:

PLEASE PAY THIS AMOUNT ➔   30.00

PLEASE MAKE CHECKS PAYABLE AND REMIT TO:

Figure 5-2 Examples of fraud include billing for services not provided, up-coding services for larger reimbursement, or down-coding (under coding) for services provided.

Infractions

Errors in billing and coding, such as accidental misfiling of claims, are handled differently from cases of deliberate fraud; however, first it must be established that an error was made. For example, suppose after a service is performed, an incorrect code is used to bill for the service, representing a simple mistake. This mistake is not deliberate fraud, but it is, of course, still an infraction, a breaking of the principles and requirements of the insurance carrier for billing and coding. It may be that this mistake is made repeatedly before the error is discovered. Under a good compliance plan, a compliance officer conducts internal random and routine audits to verify that the coding and billing is being done correctly. If the provider's compliance officer discovers an error, then the provider is required to submit documentation of these errors to the carrier and refund any monies that they have received from those errors. If this is done, the carrier sees that the provider has taken due diligence to maintain the integrity of their billing and coding practices, and no further action will be taken.

On the other hand, if it is the carrier instead who identifies the error, full audits may be initiated and possible further action and penalties may occur. Overall, the main focus in these types of cases is the intention of the provider. Was this act deliberate or intentionally misleading (and thus fraudulent)? Or did the provider and billing staff just make a mistake—that is, commit an infraction? If a case is found to be intentional, the fraudulent acts will lead to prosecution, and, as we have noted, the fines and penalties can be substantial.

Finally, an employer or healthcare organization may commit other infractions unrelated to finances or billing. For example, the Occupational Safety and Health Administration (OSHA) is a federal agency within the Department of Labor that designs, regulates, and monitors standards for employee safety. Examples of violations might include not providing an eye-wash station where needed or failing to provide appropriate means to maintain high standards of antisepsis in key treatment areas.

Abuse of Privilege

We have already seen how fraud, particularly false billing for services to gain more financial reimbursement, is an important aspect of monitoring both employees and employers in a solid compliance plan. Abuse of privilege is another. Suppose a physician strongly encourages his patients to take a particular medication with the reason being that the more prescriptions that are filled by his patients, the greater will be the physician's rewards from the drug's manufacturer. Alternatively, suppose another physician encourages her patients to seek physical and massage therapy at a particular clinic because she is part owner in that clinic—a fact she fails to share with her patients.

Both of these are examples of "kickbacks," and there are laws in place to prevent this because kickbacks are not in the best interest of the patient. Kickbacks create in a physician a bias towards promoting certain specialists, treatments, drugs, and other services or products because promotion results in personal financial gain for that physician. A body of laws called the Stark laws have been designed to maintain the integrity of the medical field and include antitrust and antikickback laws to prevent physicians from gaining financially from solicitation of services or monopolization of services.

Regulating Agencies

Besides the employer's internal compliance plan and sanctions that may be administered to employees who are guilty of violating policy/procedure, in some cases

Discussion

Using the following scenarios, determine whether disciplinary action should or should not be taken and if so what sanctions would be implemented (**NOTE:** you may not have studied the appropriate law yet, in all situations, but your ethical instincts may still lead you to the correct response):

1. A nurse is writing a prescription for a patient and signing the physician's name.
2. An employee meets a patient in the supermarket and discusses the patient's office visit earlier that day.
3. An employee is in the break room and is relating a joke that is of a sexual nature and a coworker overhearing the joke is embarrassed and offended.
4. A billing department employee discusses with a patient over the phone the possible payment plan options for the bill.
5. An employee has called in sick unexpectedly one time more than is allowed and coverage is short for that shift in the hospital.
6. A physician has already treated a patient when she realizes that the insurance policy will not be in effect for another week; she tells the front desk staff to change the date of treatment so that it will fall within the dates of coverage.
7. An employer asks an interview candidate whether or not she is planning on having more children in the near future and whether she has daycare established for her employment.
8. An employee has been given 30 days to improve work production along with additional training to aid him in his position, but after the 30-day period he is still not performing at the level of his fellow workers.
9. Sally is wearing casual dress clothing. The supervisor does not say anything to her, even though Sally is not in compliance with the dress code and other employees are held accountable to the dress code standard and are disgruntled over the situation.
10. A physician is sending all his patients to the radiological imaging center down the street; he has a partial ownership interest in the facility.

additional repercussions may be administered by the certification or licensing body, as well as other state and federal government agencies that can initiate legal charges and suspend or withdraw licensing of a provider. In addition, of course, these agencies act on federal and state mandates to monitor, regulate, correct, and sometimes take action against employers and institutions that commit errors and acts of fraud or abuse.

Each specialty is governed by their own organizations that review their qualifications, compliance, and licensure. Some of these include the following: American Medical Association (AMA); American Health Information Management Association (AHIMA); Office of the Inspector General (OIG); Centers for Medicare and Medicaid Services (CMS); Office for Civil Rights (OCR); U.S. Department of Health and Human Services (HHS); Occupational Safety and Health Administration (OSHA); nursing boards; and certification boards for all specialties and areas of allied health. We have discussed several of these in this chapter, and we encourage you to investigate more of these agencies on your own.

Each state has its own medical practice act, which provides laws that govern healthcare professionals' scope of practice and licensing requirements. Depending on the case and applicable laws, these agencies can apply sanctions that include the following, among others: loss of license, suspension of license, loss of membership to the organization, censure, licensing limitations and restrictions, required treatment (for violations involving substance abuse or psychological impairments), and requirements for further education. These would be enforced in addition to any criminal charges, fines, and sentences.

Conclusion

In the medical field, it is not just the employer and employee who need protection, but also the public. For this reason, our institutions must uphold the highest standards of care and integrity. The agencies that help regulate and monitor the healthcare field are highly specialized by profession and oversee such specialties as medical coding (AAPC), physical therapy (ABPTS), registered nursing, licensed practical nursing, clinical laboratories (CLIA), medical assisting, certified nurse anesthetists, and all areas of medicine that are under the AMA; chiropractic medicine is governed only by state boards.

Maintaining clear and concise policies and procedures in any organization is essential to upholding good practice and quality healthcare for the patients. All individuals employed will have security in knowing and understanding their employer policies and procedures and abiding to those standards, as well as knowing and working within their scope of practice for their state. Organizations function best when employees know and understand the guidelines of what is expected of them and when there is a clear, implemented, and enforced compliance plan.

Chapter Review Questions

1. The right of an employee to have certain policies and procedures followed if he or she thinks his or her rights are in jeopardy is called
   A. utilitarianism.
   B. due process.
   C. workers' compensation.
   D. HIPAA.

2. Keeping private details such as a patient's date of birth and Social Security number is an example of
   A. autonomy.
   B. HIPAA.
   C. PHI.
   D. OSHA.

3. The most important point for an employer to remember when following disciplinary action on an employee is to
   A. follow policies and procedures designated in the office handbook.
   B. make sure all actions and follow-up interactions are documented in the personnel file.
   C. counsel the employee concerning his or her rights and options in the disciplinary process.
   D. All the above

4. The definition of OIG is
   A. Office of Investigation for the Government.
   B. Office of Inspector General.
   C. Occupational Investigative Group.
   D. Office of Internal Governing.

5. The deliberate act of misrepresentation to gain financially is
   A. abuse.
   B. fraud.
   C. sanctioning.
   D. All the above

Self-Reflection Questions

1. If you were designing an employee handbook what would be some important items you would want to be sure were included in the handbook?
2. If you were in a position of management how could you ensure compliance within your staff?
3. What areas in your own specialty/field should be approached with caution?
4. What organizations can you join to ensure that you are fully mentored and guided in your specialty?
5. What would be a situation that you might try to avoid so that you do not violate a patient's HIPAA rights?

Internet Activities

1. Using the following links, review and complete a compliance self-assessment form for a place you have worked or for an environment in which you hope to be employed. Then reflect on what this experience has shown you about expectations in your field:
    - http://www.cms.gov/Medicare/Compliance-and-Audits/Part-C-and-Part-D-Compliance-and-Audits/Downloads/Compliance-Program-Effectiveness-Self-Assessment-Questionnaire.pdf
    - http://www.opm.gov/policy-data-oversight/worklife/reference-materials/workplaceviolence.pdf
2. Investigate one or more of the following laws and write an assessment of how it relates to your particular chosen field of healthcare:
    - Health Maintenance Organization Act of 1973
    - Consolidated Omnibus Budget Reconciliation Act (COBRA) of 1985
    - Drug-Free Workplace Act of 1988
    - Fair Labor Standards Act (FLSA) of 1938
    - Family Medical Leave Act (FMLA) of 1994
    - Employee Retirement Income Security Act (ERISA) of 1974
    - Emergency Medical Treatment and Active Labor Act (EMTALA)
    - Fair Credit Reporting Act of 1971
    - Fair Debt Collection Act of 1978
    - Equal Opportunity Act of 1975
    - Americans with Disabilities Act
    - The Sherman Antitrust Act
    - The National Labor Relations Act (NLRA) of 1935

Additional Resources

http://www.chirobase.org

http://www.ncsbn.org

http://www.ama-assn.org/ama/pub/physician-resources/medical-ethics/code-medical-ethics/frequently-asked-questions.page

http://www.cms.gov

http://www.aapc.com

http://oig.hhs.gov/oei/reports/oei-01-89-00560.pdf

Chapter 6

The Medical Malpractice Lawsuit and the Trial Process

Jeanne McTeigue

Affirmative defense A defense strategy that allows the defendant (usually provider or facility) to present the argument that the patient's condition was the result of factors other than negligence on the defendant's part.

Alternative dispute resolution (ADR) The procedure for settling disputes by means other than litigation.

Arbitrator Person or persons assigned by the court to mediate in a civil suit.

Assumption of risk A legal defense that asserts that the plaintiff was aware of risks and accepted the risks associated with the activity involved.

Comparative negligence (or contributory negligence) A legal defense that proves the plaintiff's own actions, or lack of action, contributed to the damages done. In this defense, compensation for damages would not be prohibited but would be reduced on the basis of the circumstance.

Compensatory damages The awarded amount given to the plaintiff in a court case to reimburse the plaintiff for loss of income or pain and suffering.

Consent The acknowledgment of a person (usually the patient) to the risks and alternatives involved in a treatment as well as permission for the treatment to be performed. This can be in some cases a verbal consent but in the medical field is usually a written document.

Damages The actual injury or loss suffered by a defendant in a suit; usually given a monetary award by the court based on the extent of the loss or injury.

Defensive medicine The physician practice of ordering unnecessary tests and other procedures to protect the physician from lawsuits.

Denial Legal assertion of innocence; made only if all four elements of negligence are false.

Dereliction (of duty) A neglect or negligence of one's duty.

Direct cause In a negligence case, the correspondence between the dereliction of duty and the actual damage sustained by the plaintiff.

Discovery rule Law or statute that states the statute of limitations does not begin until the discovery of the diagnosis or injury.

Duty In a malpractice suit, the proof of responsibility of the parties involved.

Fraud Deliberate, intentional act to mislead for financial gain.

Good Samaritan law Law providing immunity for those who render healthcare for an emergency or disaster without reimbursement.

Informed consent Same as *consent,* but in the medical field this term becomes more detailed, listing and covering all possible risks and potential prognoses for having a treatment or procedure performed and the alternatives available.

Liable Legal responsibility for a person's own actions.

Litigious Highly inclined to sue.

Malfeasance The performance of an illegal act.

Malpractice The failure of a professional to meet the standard of conduct that a reasonable and prudent member of the same profession would exercise in similar circumstances, and results in harm.

Mediation The process by which a neutral third party who is trained in mediation techniques facilitates and assists in resolving a dispute.

Misfeasance Poor performance of a duty or action, causing damage.

Negligence The failure to use such care as a reasonably prudent and careful person would use under similar circumstances; an act of omission or failure to do what a person of ordinary prudence would have done under similar circumstances.

Nominal damages A small payment or award given by the court.

Nonfeasance A failure to perform an action when needed.

Punitive damages An award granted by the courts to punish the defendant for the damages done based on a malicious or intentional act.

Release of tortfeasor Law that asserts that once the person causing damage (the tortfeasor) is released from further liability in a previous suit's settlement, he or she cannot be held liable in a subsequent suit.

Res judicata Law that forbids suing a subsequent time for the same damages once a case has already been resolved.

Respondeat superior Legal doctrine stating that, in many circumstances, an employer is responsible for the actions of employees performed within the course of their employment.

Settlement Legal agreement that is reached between two parties in a civil matter.

Statute of limitations Defense against a tort action; requires that a claim be filed within a specific amount of time of discovering that a wrong has been committed.

Subpoena *duces tecum* A Latin phrase meaning "under penalty take it with you." Used in medicolegal matters to subpoena a provider or facility to present the defendant's file or records when appearing in court.

CHAPTER OBJECTIVES

1. Define and explain malpractice.
2. Define negligence and explain the four elements necessary to establish negligence.
3. Recognize the concept of *"respondeat superior"* and its role in malpractice cases.
4. Identify and explain the three categories of duty.
5. Outline the three categories of damages that are typically awarded in malpractice cases.
6. Describe the process of establishing a case of malpractice or negligence.
7. Define and explain defenses in malpractice cases.
8. Explain professional liability.
9. Define liability prevention strategies for both individual employees and supervisors in the healthcare setting.

Introduction

Even with the best intentions, accidents can happen and mistakes can be made. Individuals need to be responsible for their actions and should be held accountable for their mistakes, actions, and/or lack of action. This is where malpractice and negligence protect those individuals who suffer damages and/or when a death occurs attributable to negligence. This is just as true when a healthcare provider is at fault and has been negligent or made errors in the treatment of a patient.

In fact, over the years there have been many cases in which the injured parties and/or their families should have, but did not, receive the appropriate compensation for their pain, suffering, or losses because of the negligence of others. It is certainly true, for example, that a family who lost a loved one because of mesothelioma caused by asbestos exposure at work should be compensated for the loss of income and the accumulation of medical expenses caused by this disease, even though nothing will change the fact that the family or individual has the disease. In these cases, many of the victims were unaware that they were being exposed to the deadly effects of asbestos and it was many years later before the disease was discovered.

However, in our current society, the general culture has become very litigious. If there is any dispute, society has encouraged the average individual to file a suit as soon as possible. Some individuals, even aware of potential risks and possible negative outcomes or prognoses, may be looking for others to blame for their losses or damages. It does not help that every other commercial on television is an advertisement for a law firm professing expertise in litigation for compensation for damages caused by a certain drug, a job-induced injury or disease, a faulty prosthetic implant, or some type of medical device. Although there are many very legitimate cases in which compensation should and is rewarded to the injured parties, today's culture persuades many individuals to sue for any and all unwanted outcomes in medical care. In many cases, the risks and potential problems with these treatments have been discussed and explained to the patient before treatment, and therefore these are not cases of negligence or error.

Some cases do not meet the criteria for malpractice laws and are considered to be "frivolous" in an attempt to gain a nominal award. For that reason, the process does include a review of each case by an expert equally qualified as the provider (defendant) to certify that the case has "merit" and should be presented. However, even when a lawsuit does not end with an award being granted, the expense and time utilized by the courts, lawyers, and providers are still recorded as a case filed against that provider.

Thus, the vicious cycle begins. Providers feel forced to practice defensive medicine, sometimes ordering unnecessary tests or procedures just to protect themselves, to assert that they did all they could for a patient; and then the rates of insurance are increased because of the amount of cost incurred; this, in turn, means that patients have to pay higher premiums and deductibles for health insurance. Similarly, physicians/providers have to pay higher malpractice insurance as a result of cases filed against them. Costs for services in the medical field must increase to cover the expense of the insurances, and so the cycle continues.

The good news is that our court systems do have some tools that attempt to find a balance—that is, both to protect the victims from negligence and wrongful deaths and to try to protect the providers/defendants (mainly by requiring plaintiffs to establish proof of negligence and cause). Many cases of malpractice are initiated that do not end in trial but in negotiations and settlements outside of court. Because of the expense and the exposure, many facilities and practices may offer settlements just to avoid lengthy legal processes and expense. Settlements can reach agreement through an arbitrator or mediation process. In cases with clear negligence, often these will be handled before trial. It is dependent on the defense attorney and the malpractice insurance carrier to decide, in consultation with the defendant, whether an agreement can be arranged before actual trial.

Finally, most states instill a statute of limitations. This type of law varies among states, but its purpose is to limit the amount of time after the injury or discovery of the injury (based on the discovery rule) for the plaintiff to file a lawsuit. In other words, after a certain number of years, it can become simply too late to file a suit.

Malpractice and Negligence

So what exactly is malpractice? Malpractice occurs when a party (or parties) responsible for the care or treatment of an individual either acts or fails to act, resulting in damages and/or direct losses to the patient or individual. The categories of malpractice are based on the duty of the parties responsible. After establishing responsibility or duty (called *feasance*), malpractice may be divided into subcategories of *malfeasance, nonfeasance,* and *misfeasance.* The most common area of malpractice is negligence. Thus the court speaks about negligence in terms of duty, dereliction of duty, direct cause, and damages. These four elements must be established in order to pursue a case based on negligence.

Recent legislation under review could enact updates to malpractice laws in the following two areas:

1. New legislation could make it easier to obtain a certificate of merit, meaning that a case could be reviewed by a heathcare provider (not necessarily one of the same specialty or experience), allowing for cases to be heard that may not have previously been considered "merited."
2. New legislation being considered could increase the burden of proof on the plaintiff from the legal term of "preponderance of evidence" (standard 99.9%) in malpractice cases to the legal term of "clear and convincing."

 What If?

Bob is working as an orderly at ABC Medical Center in the evening while going to school during the day. One evening as Bob is entering the hospital, he hears a noise from around the corner and then the sound of squealing brakes. Bob looks around the corner of the building but does not see anything except the taillights of a fast moving car as it turns onto a side street. Bob shrugs his shoulders and goes into the hospital. Two days later he is reading the newspaper and sees a story about a young man who died two nights ago after being dumped outside ABC Medical Center.

Bob realizes that he might have seen the car that dumped the young man, but he does not remember seeing any people around because it was dark and there are several shrubs on that side of the building. Bob is worried that he might be involved in this situation after reading that the family is threatening to sue the hospital and anyone else who was "there" when their family member died.

---

1. What should Bob do?
2. Could the family sue Bob for medical malpractice or negligence?

In the meantime, however, current cases of negligence must prove the four elements of negligence: duty, dereliction of duty, direct cause, and damages.

Duty

To establish that a healthcare provider defendant had a duty, the plaintiff must be able to prove the affirmative for the following types of questions:

1. Was the individual or facility (provider/defendant) responsible to the patient in the situation?
2. Who are the responsible parties involved?

Respondeat superior

So, who is responsible in a malpractice case?

Part of determining the responsible parties involves a concept referred to as *respondeat superior,* which means *let the master answer.* Harry S. Truman had a sign on the oval office desk that read "the buck stops here." In other words the individual with the highest license or training and/or the owner or highest authority of an organization is ultimately the individual responsible for the actions of their employees or subordinate workers (Figure 6-1). This does not exclude a healthcare provider from responsibility but demands that the person most responsible is aware of and provides training and education to the subordinate staff to ensure the adherence to policies, procedures, and scope of practice. As an example, if a respiratory care therapist is sued for actions that harm a patient, the physician and his or her employer (hospital) can also be sued. The employer can be sued on the basis both that the employer had control, or should have had control, over the actions of the *respiratory care therapist* and that the *therapist* was working in the course and scope of his or her employment.

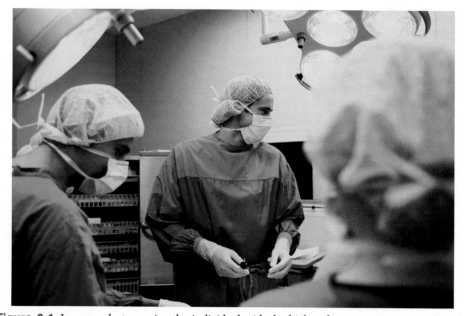

Figure 6-1 In *respondeat superior,* the individual with the highest license or training and/or the owner or highest authority of an organization is ultimately the individual responsible for actions of their subordinate workers.

Next, the courts usually require application of the "prudent person rule," which dictates that the same type of provider in the same area (geographically) would provide the same service or duty in the same situation. For instance, an exam performed by any dermatologist in a given area would and should include the same basic areas examined. Another example would be that all nurses in a given area would be expected to cross-reference drug interactions and allergies before administering a medication. These are examples of what a patient should expect from a provider as a general standard for the patient's care.

What If?

As a nursing assistant, you are assigned to a different unit to work with the nursing staff. The nurse you are assigned to is the best friend of your sister. She is often missing from the unit and you cannot find her to report on your patients.

You report to the nurse that the blood pressure is high for Mrs. Nicholson and that she claims her head hurts. After reporting this information to the nurse, the nurse disappears. A half hour later, you walk into the room and Mrs. Nicholson is drooling and has paralysis on the left side of her body. The nurse implores you not to tell the nurse manager that you reported an elevated blood pressure and headache because she is on probation.

1. Who is responsible in this scenario?
2. Are the four elements of negligence present in this scenario?
3. Are there issues that can affect the licenses of the healthcare providers?

Categories of Duty

Now that we have established what the law means by "duty," we will look more closely at the three categories of duty (or *feasance*):

- Malfeasance—an intentional action or performance of an illegal or wrongful act. An example might be a provider working outside their scope of practice (which can vary among states).
- Nonfeasance—a failure to perform an action that should have been taken. An example would be a nurse who did *not* ask about known allergies but should have questioned the patient.
- Misfeasance—a poor performance of an action causing damage. A mistake or poor technique causes injury or pain to the patient as an example.

Discussion

1. What is the difference between the types of feasance?
2. Give examples for each type of feasance as it may pertain to the medical field.

Dereliction of Duty

To establish dereliction of duty, both sides must address the following question: Was the defendant in violation of performing the established duty? For example, if it was expected that a nurse should not administer any medication without first verifying patient allergies and the nurse failed to follow this procedure and administered the medication, this would constitute dereliction of the nurse's duty.

Direct Cause

If it is proven that the defendant is responsible (has a duty in the situation) and it is proven that this defendant did not perform his or her duty, the plaintiff will next need to prove that the damages or losses incurred by the patient were directly related to that negligent act. Using the previous example, if the patient had an allergic reaction to a medication that was administered and the nurse had not checked for patient allergies, then this would be a direct cause of the patient suffering the allergic reaction.

Damages

Once the other areas of negligence are established then the court must determine the damages that were caused by the direct dereliction of duty. Again using the preceding example, if the patient suffered an allergic reaction that required hospital services and caused that patient pain and suffering, these would all be considered damages directly related to the negligence of that nurse.

In this example, the negligence is fairly evident and straightforward, but in many cases there are other influencing factors that cause problems the patient might suffer. You may have a patient who has other chronic conditions that can affect the healing or recovery for that patient and therefore could be a contributing factor to the damages suffered.

For damages to be recovered in any case, all four elements of negligence need to be proven. Once this occurs then damages can be awarded to the injured party and can include recovery for any permanent disability, loss of employment or wages, pain and suffering, medical or hospital expenses, permanent mental disability, future loss of earnings if unable to return to employment, and loss of enjoyment attributable to injuries and/or disabilities suffered.

Depending on the feasance that is determined, these fines and/or reimbursements can be different between states but usually fall into the following categories:

- Compensatory damages—financial losses based on actual income or expenses, for example. Recovery of these losses can be awarded.
- Punitive damages—awards usually based on an intentional act or wrongful act that was performed and used as a punishment for the wrongful act. This usually amounts to a large sum of money.
- Nominal damages—small awards given when no major damages were suffered. However, the injured party still had a violation of their rights or a negligent act was committed.

Finally, if the injured party were to expire, the family may be awarded sums of money as a settlement in a wrongful death case. The laws addressing wrongful death suits vary among states, with some states setting a maximum limit.

Establishing a Case

As important as it is to show the elements of negligence in such cases, the plaintiff (patient) usually has the duty to prove these elements with the "preponderance of evidence." In other words, responsibility rests on the plaintiff to prove the case, as

Relate to Practice

A patient is admitted to the hospital with gallstones and needs to have his gallbladder removed. This is considered an emergency surgery because of the position of the stones and the level of patient pain. The patient also suffers from type 2 diabetes that is not well controlled. The patient undergoes surgery and the gallbladder is found to be gangrenous; the gallbladder is removed but the patient suffers from jaundice following surgery. After follow-up testing, it is determined that the bile duct from the gallbladder was damaged during the emergency surgery and the patient needs another surgical procedure to repair its damage.

1. How would the components of negligence be met in this case?
2. Are there any other mitigating factors involved?

opposed to the defendant. An exception to this would be if the case is decided by a judge (pretrial) to be *res ipsa loquitur,* which means "the thing speaks for itself." This would have to be established by the plaintiff pretrial and ruled on by a judge in most states. *Res ipsa loquitur* means that there is clear evidence of negligence and there was no possible way that the patient (plaintiff) could have effected a different outcome or contributed to the damages or injury. It also indicates that there is clear proof that the defendant had the responsibility (duty) to the patient and that the injury would not and could not have occurred without the negligence of the defendant. For example, a physician performs an operation on the right arm instead of the left. In these cases, the burden of proof then falls on the defendant to prove there was no negligence.

Defenses for Malpractice

Before a case actually goes to a full trial, both parties may agree to try an **alternative dispute resolution (ADR)**, using mediation and an arbitrator. This can be a successful way to expedite the processes and also aid in maintaining the expense and time for all parties involved since malpractice cases that go to trial are known to be an extremely lengthy process.

In addition, some technical defenses can prevent a case from ever going to trial. For example, most states have a *statute of limitations,* as we have mentioned earlier in this chapter, which means that the plaintiff has a limited number of years after discovery of damages in which to file a suit. After that, it is simply too late. Similarly, under *res judicata,* the patient cannot sue a second time for the same damages once a case has already been resolved. Similar to this is the **release of tortfeasor,** which asserts that if the person causing damage (the tortfeasor) is released from further liability in a previous suit's settlement, he or she cannot be held liable in a subsequent suit.

However, if the case does go to trial, there are several key types of defense for malpractice suits.

Denial

If allegations are entirely false, the defendant may assert his or her innocence. This defense can only be used if *all* aspects of the complaint are false. If some are true, then the defendant instead will address those elements of negligence that are missing or false.

Affirmative Defense

In this form of malpractice defense, the defendant asserts that the outcome was contributed to or possibly caused by other factors beyond the alleged negligence. In these defenses it is a denial of negligence. For example, a patient may ignore pre- or post-treatment instructions, or refuse to comply with follow-up requirements. The patient may also have lifestyle factors that contributed to the negative outcome. These forms of affirmative defense are referred to as contributory negligence or comparative negligence (see following discussion).

Emergency Care

Affirmative defense is also frequently used in emergency care. One of the highest risk areas for malpractice cases exists in emergency medicine. There is no previous relationship with the patient and generally no prior treatment known by the provider. The physician may have very limited history for the patient and limited knowledge of past medical, family, and social histories. In an emergency treatment, the emergency department staff will usually verify vital information, such as allergies to medications (when patient or family are able to provide it), but the condition may be such that there would be very limited time to obtain full details. Similar information and time limitations exist in other high-risk situations, including in the intensive care unit, during emergency transplantation, or during neonatal crises and labor and delivery.

Good Samaritan Laws

Medical professionals who respond in good faith in an emergency may also be protected under the Good Samaritan laws. It is a legal and ethical responsibility of trained individuals to assist in emergency situations if they are a witness to such situations. In these cases, the patient needs emergency help, but may have conditions that he or she is not able to communicate and that contribute to complications or further injury. For example, in the case of witnessing an automobile accident or a person choking in a restaurant, the trained person should not just pass by or walk away from the emergency, and yet the person could be legally vulnerable because he or she lacks full patient information. For this reason, states have come to recognize that healthcare professionals need protection from liability and litigation in such cases. In the past, physicians, nurses, and other trained professionals often failed to aid an injured person because of fear of possible lawsuits. As a result, these Good Samaritan laws have been developed to protect against litigation in emergencies. As long as a provider or trained professional is not working under their employment at the time, they are covered under the Good Samaritan law and cannot be sued for malpractice (Figure 6-2).

Comparative Negligence or Contributory Negligence

In this form of defense, the defendant shows that the action or inaction of the plaintiff was a contributing factor in the damages that were incurred. For example, suppose a patient suffers from complications from a surgical procedure that resulted in damages or further injury, but the patient did not follow up with the physician or notify the physician immediately that there was a problem. In such a case, the defendant (physician) could argue that the lack of follow-up action on the patient's part was at least partially responsible for the damages suffered.

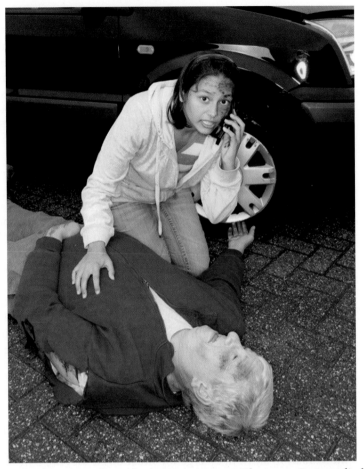

Figure 6-2 A *Good Samaritan law*, active in most states, provides immunity to medical professionals who provide healthcare in an emergency without reimbursement or without proper facilities available.

Relate to Practice

A middle-aged male presented at the emergency department of a local hospital with stroke-like symptoms. After a thorough examination, a vascular surgeon was assigned to operate on the patient. Following a brief postsurgical hospital stay, the surgeon released the patient with instructions to take daily doses of the prescription drug Coumadin and ordered a follow-up examination to monitor the effect of the drug.

The patient failed to comply and did not attend his follow-up appointment. In fact, he never again consulted with the surgeon who prescribed the medication. Over the next 12 months, the patient had prescriptions for Coumadin refilled. During this time the patient changed pharmacy locations at least twice and had the script transferred. The last pharmacy accidentally recorded the date of the prescription as the date of transfer. This resulted in the pharmacy refilling the Coumadin beyond the 1-year date, at which time the prescription would have expired. The patient died from internal bleeding caused by "long-term Coumadin use." The executor of the patient's estate brought suit against the surgeon and the pharmacy.

1. Was the surgeon or the pharmacy, or both, negligent?
2. Was the patient guilty of contributory negligence?

Assumption of Risk

This form of defense relies on accurate documentation, particularly in two key areas: First and foremost, before any procedure, a patient is required to sign a document of informed consent. The informed consent lists and details all possible risks involved in a treatment/procedure and possible outcomes or complications. It lists clearly any medications or behaviors that a patient should avoid before the procedure (such as no eating or drinking 12 hours before the procedure), as well as restrictions and responsibilities that should be followed through final follow-up visits. Second, the informed consent will also detail the possible ramifications or consequences of not having the procedure.

In assumption of risk, the medical record is the best defense, if documented properly, accurately, and completely. The records should show the entire series of events leading up to the point of the alleged negligence. The patient (plaintiff) has "duty" to the provider (defendant) that plays an important role in the diagnosis, treatment, and prognosis for any patient. Examples include honesty in giving medical history and related family histories as well as compliance with the prescribed treatment and/or recommended follow-up instructions (and this includes lifestyle changes such as diet and exercise, for example).

In most cases, a subpoena *duces tecum* (Latin phrase meaning "under penalty take it with you") would be issued by the courts to the defendant to bring the physical chart to court when appearing to testify.

What If?

A patient is seen by a gastroenterologist and it is recommended that the patient undergo a colonoscopy procedure for diagnostic purposes. The physician reviews the risks of having the procedure done as well as the consequences of not having the procedure performed. The patient signs an informed consent form, and the medical assistant/nurse reviews the preparation instructions the patient should follow before the procedure as well as other details. In the instructions, it is clearly noted that the patient should stop taking any medications, such as aspirin, that can cause bleeding problems at least 7 days before the surgery. However, the patient continues to take a single 81-mg dose of aspirin each evening, dismissing the possible complication that this could have during the procedure. On the day of the procedure, the physician records that the patient has confirmed following all preoperative instructions. Afterward, the patient has a bleeding complication in response to the procedure, is hospitalized for this complication, and sues the physician.

1. What example of defense is this case?
2. Who is responsible in this case?
3. Was the provider/physician negligent?

Professional Liability

Under the *respondeat superior* doctrine (Latin for "Let the master answer") the physician or provider would be liable for the actions of anyone under their employ. In cases of malpractice, if a nurse or medical assistant, for example, does cause harm or damage while performing a venipuncture on a patient, then the medical assistant or nurse could or would be named in the suit, but also the physician or facility would be named as a responsible party. All parties involved would be liable for their contribution in the case, but the one held most responsible is the highest licensed of the practice and/ or the employer of the individual named that caused the harm and/or showed negligence.

Professional liability insurance, including malpractice coverage, is carried by providers and facilities as well as many other allied healthcare providers, such as nurses, medical assistants, and technicians. Medical liability insurance usually covers malpractice not only for the providers but also for the employees (as long as they are working within their legal scope of practice) and the premises as well. Not unlike a homeowner's policy, this would cover any liability if an injury or accident occurred on the premises attributable to a fault in the condition of the premises (e.g., if a patient fell on the front steps of the office because of ice or a broken step).

Prevention of Liability and Malpractice

In the healthcare field professionals are dealing every day with the well-being and lives of their patients. It is vitally important that providers always remind themselves that the patient is most important and beware of vulnerabilities. Many times arrogance, burn-out, or lack of knowledge and experience can lead to errors and negligence. Mistakes in judgment and errors occur and those responsible must be held accountable.

The following are some ways to help prevent malpractice:

- Always working within your scope of practice
- Never promising a cure to a patient
- Carefully identifying and confirming identification of a patient before treatment
- Always verifying allergies of a patient
- Documenting **every** patient encounter
- Staying current in the field
- Treating all patients with dignity and respect
- Working only within your job description and knowing the policies and procedures of the employer

Role of the Risk Management Supervisor

In the field of medicine the individual who takes steps to reduce liability may be a nurse manager, a unit manager, an office manager, or a physician. For simplification, let us use the example of an office manager. These individuals aid in protecting the provider or *respondeat superior* from liability. The risk management supervisor's duties would include monitoring all aspects of prevention of malpractice and guarding the practice against issues of fraud and abuse (Figure 6-3). The practice would have in place a compliance plan and policies and procedures that must be followed to ensure that both clinically and administratively the practice is covered. This should include in-services and training for all staff to ensure that everyone is up to date on the newest knowledge in clinical practice and in billing and coding. All checks and balances should be in place to regulate and monitor these areas on a regular basis. Finally, every practice must have documented policies, a current compliance plan, enforced job descriptions specific for each employee, up-to-date education and in-services, and an effective system of checks and balances to protect all areas of the practice from litigation and liability.

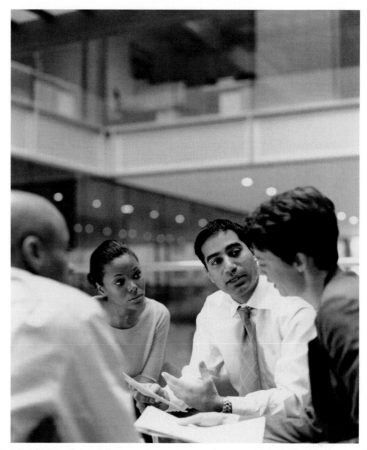

Figure 6-3 The duties of the risk management supervisor would include monitoring all aspects of prevention of malpractice and guarding the practice against issues of fraud and abuse.

Duties of a Risk Management Supervisor

Specific duties within the primary role of a supervisor or administrator fall largely into the areas of safety, communication, and documentation, consisting in large part in the following capacities:

Safety of Staff and Patients
- Implementing a quality improvement (QI) plan to keep all practices at current health field standards
- Training of staff and regularly assessing skill competencies, credentialing, and continuing education, including appropriate training in operation of equipment
- Maintaining appropriate safety standards of the premises and physical environment
- Monitoring safe handling of drugs on site as well as hazardous materials
- Enforcing OSHA guidelines and other federal and state regulations and credentialing
- Ensuring that appropriate liability insurance is acquired and maintained
- Overseeing sterilization of materials and equipment
- Maintaining safety standards of equipment
- Regularly reviewing the facility's disaster plan

Communication
- Ensuring that all staff members are current on the policies and procedures that pertain to their roles in the practice
- Ensuring that all HIPAA confidentiality is safeguarded in both electronic and physical areas of the practice
- Communicating with patients to ensure that the practice is running well and that patients' needs are being met (e.g., patient phone calls are being responded to in a timely manner; patients feel that they are being heard and that the staff responds to them in a caring fashion; staff is adhering to high standards of professionalism)
- Overseeing all written communications for the patients to ensure that all are up to date, available for clinical staff, and regularly used (e.g., patient education materials, preoperative instructions, and consent forms)

Documentation
- Establishing and implementing the forms required for patient encounters, including informed consent, and for billing
- Providing a means for staff to ensure that all communication with a client—including verbal and phone exchanges—is documented
- Keeping records of cancellations and no-shows, as well as recording appropriate follow-up and patient compliance incidents with both appointments and instructions
- Double-checking all charges and coding; verifying all monies collected for accuracy to avoid errors in the patients' balances and to avoid errors to the insurance carriers
- Scheduling regular audits of billing and coding, both randomly and routinely, to correct any problems quickly and efficiently

All these areas are vital to prevention both of malpractice issues and of fraud and abuse or HIPAA violations. In any facility, practice, or organization the role of these individuals is paramount to the viability of the practice itself and the safety and care of the patients.

Finally, physicians can reduce their own liability risks by: (a) ensuring that they obtain adequate diagnostic results before beginning a patient's course of treatment; (b) double-checking dosage and medication for a patient; (c) avoiding unnecessary use of toxic or risky tests or treatments whenever possible; and (d) making an effort to have an assistant present during examination, preferably of the same gender as the patient when possible.

Conclusion

In medicine there is always a chance that errors will occur and if injuries occur as a result, the responsible parties should be held accountable. No one in the healthcare field wants to make these errors, so the best solution is to have a proactive attitude and to have systems in place to guard against and prevent issues from arising.

Chapter Review Questions

1. The four components of negligence are
   A. duty, dereliction of duty, damages, and direct cause.
   B. duty, differences, damages, and direct cause.
   C. duty, dereliction, direct cause, and danger to others.
   D. duty, direct cause, deletion, and damages.

2. An example of a high-risk area in the healthcare field for malpractice would be in
   A. the emergency department.
   B. administration.
   C. laboratory facilities.
   D. the radiology department.

3. What would be an important element in a malpractice case?
   A. What the physician thinks is right
   B. What the hospital thinks happened
   C. What the patient feels is fair
   D. What the documentation reflects happened

4. Who can be named in a malpractice case?
   A. Only a physician
   B. Only a hospital
   C. Only the person who directly allegedly injured the patient
   D. All parties who were involved in the case where the alleged injury occurred

5. The discovery rule applies to
   A. the patient's ability to work.
   B. the first time an injury occurs in a facility.
   C. the discovery of a new treatment for an illness.
   D. the statute of limitations for suing for an injury or illness.

Self-Reflection Questions

1. How do you protect yourself from negligence or errors in your work?
2. Would it be necessary or advisable for you to examine your own liability insurance policy?
3. What things can you do to ensure the safety and well-being of your patients?
4. What organizations can you join, both periodicals and Internet sites, to keep current in your field?

Internet Activities

1. Access the following article regarding new legislation on malpractice and write a summary of the article: http://articles.courant.com/2013-03-29/health/hc-er-mal practice-bill-20130329_1_malpractice-suits-public-health-committee-change-malpractice-law.
2. Research the scope of practice for your profession in your state to ensure you know the individual state guidelines for your field.

Additional Resources

www.legalinfo.com/content/medical-malpractice/defenses-to-medical-malpractice.html
http://blog.vascularsurgeryexpertwitness.com/files/defending_med_malpractice.pdf
www.abpla.org/what-is-malpractice
www.thedoctors.com
www.medicalmalpracticehelp.com
www.cms.gov
www.ama-assn.org
www.findlaw.com

Chapter 7

Intentional and Quasi-Intentional Torts

Christopher Lee

Assault A threat or attempt to inflict offensive physical contact or bodily harm on a person that puts the person in immediate danger of or in apprehension of such harm or contact.

Battery Bodily harm or unlawful touching of another. In the medical field, treating a patient without consent is considered battery.

Breach of confidentiality The public revelation of confidential or privileged information without an individual's consent.

Consent The acknowledgment of one (usually the patient) to the risks and alternatives involved in a treatment and the permission for the treatment to be performed. This can be in some cases a verbal consent but in the medical field is usually a written document.

Defamation Any intentional false communication, either written or spoken, that harms a person's reputation; decreases the respect, regard, or confidence in which a person is held; or induces disparaging, hostile, or disagreeable opinions or feelings against a person.

False imprisonment Restraint of a person so as to impede his or her liberty without justification or consent.

Implied consent Consent that is not expressly granted by a person, but rather inferred from a person's actions and the facts and circumstances of a particular situation.

Informed consent Same as consent but, in the medical field, more detailed, listing and covering all possible risks and potential prognoses for having a treatment or procedure done and the alternatives available.

Intent The willful decision to bring about a prohibited consequence.

Intentional infliction of emotional distress Type of conduct that deliberately causes severe emotional trauma to the victim.

Intentional tort A category of torts that describes a civil wrong resulting from an intentional act on the part of another person or entity.

Invasion of privacy The wrongful intrusion into private affairs with which the perpetrator or the public has no concern.

Liability Obligations under law arising from civil actions or torts.

Libel Written, printed, or other visual communication that harms another person's reputation.

Malpractice The failure of a professional to meet the standard of conduct that a reasonable and prudent member of their profession would exercise in similar circumstances; results in harm.

Negligence The failure to use such care as a reasonably prudent and careful person would use under similar circumstances; an act of omission or failure to do what a person of ordinary prudence would have done under similar circumstances.

Quasi-intentional tort A voluntary act that directly causes damage to a person's privacy or emotional well-being, but without the intent to injure or to cause distress.

Sexual assault Any type of sexual activity unwanted or unwelcomed by a person.

Slander Spoken or verbal communication in which one person discusses another in terms that harm the person's reputation.

Tort A wrongful act, not including a breach of contract or trust, that results in injury to another's person, property, reputation, or the like, and for which the injured party is entitled to compensation.

Trespass An unlawful intrusion that interferes with one's person, property (called "chattels"), or land.

CHAPTER OBJECTIVES

1. Discuss the nature of intentional and quasi-intentional torts and describe how they differ from negligence or strict liability.
2. Discuss the necessary intent needed to commit an intentional or quasi-intentional tort.
3. List and describe specific types of intentional torts.
4. Explain the importance of consent.
5. Analyze defenses for specific types of intentional torts.
6. List and describe specific types of quasi-intentional torts.
7. Analyze defenses for specific types of quasi-intentional torts.
8. Determine insurance coverage for intentional and quasi-intentional torts.

Introduction

In day-to-day practice, healthcare professionals confront situations in which they must perform invasive, sometimes painful, and often-humiliating procedures on their patients. Under different circumstances, these actions can give rise to legal actions against the healthcare professional. Although most healthcare professionals are concerned with negligence or malpractice actions, there is another area of law where potential liability rests. It is the area known as intentional and quasi-intentional torts (Box 7-1).

Definition of a Tort

A tort is a civil wrong other than breach of contract. The word *tort* is derived from an Old Norman word meaning "wrong." It involves harm against a person, whereas a crime is harm against the state. For example, someone steals your purse. You file a complaint with the police, and the police arrest John Jones for the crime of theft. When Jones goes to court, the case is titled *State v. John Jones*. The state brings the action because a crime is deemed a harm against the peace and tranquility of all persons in the state, not just the victim.

If a tort is committed, however, an individual brings the case against another individual. The state does not have an interest in seeing that you are paid money damages for any loss you sustained. In the preceding example, you can bring a civil action

BOX 7-1
Intentional and Quasi-Intentional Torts

Intentional tort: A civil wrongdoing that requires intentional interference with one's person, reputation, or property.

Assault: Placing someone in immediate fear or apprehension of a harmful or noxious touching without consent; the person must be aware that you are about to touch him or her.

Battery: A harmful or offensive touching of another without consent or without a legally justifiable reason; without consent or absent an emergency, any touching of a patient can be battery.

False imprisonment: The unlawful detention of a person where he or she is deprived of personal liberty of movement against his or her will and without any authority to detain. To be falsely imprisoned, a person must be confined within a specific area against his or her will; he or she must be confined by physical, chemical, or emotional means and/or by physical force or threat of physical force; and he or she must be aware of the confinement.

Intentional infliction of emotional distress: Conduct is outrageous and beyond the bounds of common decency. Insulting behavior is not enough; the actions must be egregious.

Trespass to land: Occurs when a person, without the consent of the owner, enters on another's land or causes anyone or anything to enter the land. Harm to the land is not required, but without harm, damages are usually nominal.

Quasi-intentional torts: Include defamation, invasion of privacy, and breach of confidentiality. *Quasi* means "resembling"–these types of torts resemble intentional torts but are different because they are based on speech.

Defamation: A false statement or communication that a speaker knows or should know is false and that is published to third parties and damages a person's reputation. *Truth* is an absolute defense to defamation. Libel is written defamation. Slander is oral defamation.

Invasion of privacy: Unjustifiable intrusion on another's right of privacy by:
Appropriating his or her name or likeness
Unreasonably interfering with his or her seclusion
Publishing private facts
Placing the person in a false light
Invasion of privacy differs from defamation. In most instances, the information is true but is information that a person wants to keep private. Although defamation causes injury to reputation, invasion of privacy causes injury to feelings.

Breach of confidentiality: A legal and ethical issue. The code of ethics of allied health personnel must emphasize that healthcare professionals must safeguard patients' right to privacy by judiciously protecting confidential information.

against John Jones for any loss you sustained in the theft of your purse. In such an action, you seek money damages for the loss.

Almost all torts can be crimes, but most crimes are not torts. If prison is the penalty, then the action is a crime. If money damages are the penalty, then the action is a tort.

There are four types of torts: **negligence,** *intentional torts, quasi-intentional torts,* and *strict liability.* You may recall that negligence was discussed in Chapter 6, where we established that cases of negligence must prove the four elements of negligence: duty, dereliction of duty, damages, and direct cause. Overall, then, the essence of negligence is a breach of established standards of care, whereas the essence of strict liability is the relationship to or ownership of the thing that caused harm. Because we have already discussed negligence in Chapter 6, we can turn our attention to intentional and quasi-intentional torts.

Intentional Torts

The major intentional torts are assault, battery, false imprisonment, intentional infliction of emotional distress, and, in specific areas of nursing such as home care, trespass. Broadly defined, intentional torts require that there be an intentional interference with an individual's person, reputation, or property.

Intent

To determine intent, we do not necessarily have to establish that the accused individual had a desire to bring about harm or injury to a person (Figure 7-1). Instead, it is enough to be able to demonstrate that any reasonable person would or should be substantially certain that specific results will follow from his or her actions. In other words, suppose you walk behind a healthcare provider into a hospital hallway just as he pulls a tray from the dinner cart and it hits you; in this case, there is no intent to harm you, and no intentional tort is committed. However, if that same healthcare provider takes the

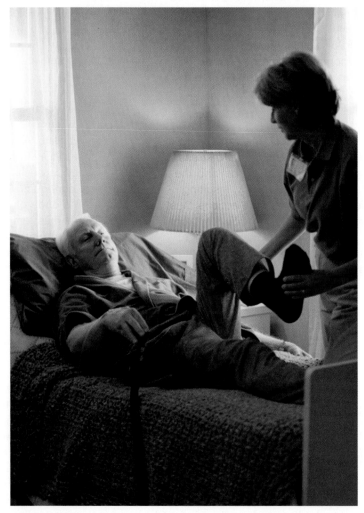

Figure 7-1 To determine intent, we do not necessarily have to establish that the accused individual had a desire to cause harm or injury to a person.

tray and throws it across the room at a patient's bed so that it hits the patient, then he knew or should have known that the action of throwing a tray was likely to hit someone and cause injury. That knowledge is sufficient to assert that the worker has demonstrated the intent necessary to commit an intentional tort of assault and battery.

Intent may also be transferred. For example, suppose you intend to shoot person A, but you miss and shoot person B instead. Even though you have no intent to harm person B, your intent to harm person A is transferred, and the law deems that you had the intent to harm person B. It is a rule of law that "intent follows the bullet." Although transferred intent does not often occur in the medical setting, if a healthcare provider gives the wrong patient an injection, the provider can be liable for battery and negligence, even though he or she has no intent to harm that patient or any conscious desire to administer the injection to the wrong patient.

To be liable for an intentional tort, a person must meet all elements of the tort. If any one element is missing, then no tort has been committed. Each of the specific torts mentioned previously—assault, battery, false imprisonment, intentional infliction of emotional distress—requires the presence of specific elements. We next examine each of these torts, and the conditions each must meet to be defined.

Assault

The first type of tort, *assault,* means placing someone in immediate fear or apprehension of harmful or unpleasant touching without the person's consent. To commit an assault, the person must be aware, or fearful, that you are about to touch him or her.

For example, a patient is in bed crying and becomes hysterical. The home health aide caring for the patient becomes increasingly anxious and upset as a result of the patient's behavior. The aide raises her hand over her head and threatens to strike the patient. The aide does not have to say anything to the patient; instead, raising her hand as if to strike is enough. If the patient sees the aide raising her hand and cringes to protect herself, then the patient is put in imminent fear of battery, and the aide has thus committed an assault.

If, on the other hand, the patient is crying into her pillow and does not see the aide raise her hand to strike, then the patient is not put in fear of an imminent battery, and no assault is committed.

Usually, however, an assault precedes a battery, and the two torts are often grouped together. Keep in mind, however, that they are two separate torts.

Battery

A *battery* is harmful or offensive touching of another without his or her consent or without a legally justifiable reason. Without the consent of the patient, or absent an emergency, any touching of a patient can be battery.

Committing battery does not mean you try to maliciously hurt or strike a person. Although hitting, spitting at, kicking, or slapping a patient are all, of course, forms of battery, it can be more subtle than that. Any touching, such as inserting an intravenous device, may be battery if done without the consent of the person or without a legally justifiable reason. In addition, you do not need to even touch a patient to commit battery; instead, if you just touch something in close proximity to the person without his or her consent, then battery is committed. For example, if a patient wants to leave the hospital against medical advice, and as the healthcare provider, you grab her purse or suitcase from her hand, even if it is just to get her to listen to you, you have committed battery. Even though your intent may have been noble (i.e., protecting her health by keeping her in the hospital), it is still, nevertheless, battery.

Discussion
What are your thoughts on a healthcare provider being sued for battery when the provider's actions were in the best interests of the patient?

Consent: A Primary Defense Against Battery

As we have just seen, *battery* is any offensive touching, or any touching (even therapeutic contact), done without permission or in the absence of an emergency situation. In the normal treatment setting, then, all patients admitted to a hospital are required to sign a general consent. This general consent is for medical care and treatment and grants permission for other employees of the hospital to "touch" the patient, as needed, in a therapeutic manner. Do not confuse this *general consent* with an informed consent to surgery or to other invasive procedures. Although the failure to obtain an informed consent may lead to an action in medical negligence, the consent necessary to avoid battery is the permission to touch the person.

Yet, consent is not automatic protection from charges of battery. A medical *battery* can be committed in specific situations in which there is consent to perform one particular procedure, but you perform another instead. At the cornerstone of this theory is the decision of the brilliant jurist Justice Benjamin Cardozo, who wrote in 1914: "Every human being of adult years and sound mind has a right to determine what shall be done with his own body, and a surgeon who performs an operation without his patient's consent commits an assault for which he is liable in damages."

Although you may think that no person would perform a procedure other than the one authorized, several cases are instructive. In *Pizzaloto v. Wilson,* the patient gave consent for the surgeon to perform exploratory surgery to accomplish lysis of adhesions and fulguration of endometriosis. During the abdominal surgery, the physician noted that the plaintiff's reproductive organs had sustained severe damage. He determined that she was in fact sterile and proceeded to remove both her uterus and ovaries.

When the plaintiff awoke from surgery, she was upset with the actions taken by the physician. In ruling in her favor, the court ruled that the plaintiff was entitled to recover damages because there was no emergency present and the surgeon committed battery. The court awarded her $10,000. A similar example is seen in the case of *Guin v. Sison,* in which the court awarded $1000 to a postmenopausal woman who had her left fallopian tube and ovary removed without consent during the course of colon surgery.

Female patients are not the only ones who need be concerned. In a recent Pennsylvania case, the plaintiff had sought the defendant's assistance for treatment of premature ejaculation. After conservative treatment gave only temporary relief, the defendant suggested a surgery to remove plaque from the plaintiff's penis. Upon awakening from surgery, the plaintiff was given a warranty card by the nurse for the penile implant the defendant had inserted during surgery. It was undisputed that no consent was given for the implant. While the trial court originally dismissed the claim because the plaintiff did not have an expert witness, the appeals court reversed and ordered the trial court to proceed with the case.

In each of the examples given, the physicians' defense was based on their claim that they were protecting their patients from the need for a second surgery. Even if true, and even though the physicians performed both surgeries skillfully, the courts still held that the decision to undergo specific surgery is the plaintiff's, and absent an emergency, a physician cannot exceed the scope of the patient's consent. If the physician does so, he or she commits battery.

Physicians are not the only ones who commit medical battery. Consider the facts of *Roberson v. Provident House,* in which the plaintiff, a quadriplegic, was admitted to the defendant's nursing home. The plaintiff wore an external condom catheter, but the nursing staff obtained an order to insert an internal Foley catheter as needed. The order was obtained because occasionally problems developed with the condom catheter and the patient leaked urine. The physician did not discuss the insertion of a Foley catheter with the plaintiff, and the plaintiff was unaware that the order was written.

On two separate occasions the Foley catheter was inserted over the objections of the plaintiff, despite his repeated requests to have the catheter removed. After the second insertion, when the plaintiff complained bitterly each shift, one nurse, who was tired of the plaintiff's complaints, jerked the catheter out, causing a discharge of blood and pus. The court found the nursing staff and their employer liable for battery. The plaintiff was awarded $25,000.

This case teaches several lessons. First and foremost, if your patient refuses to allow you to perform a procedure, **stop.** Second, if the patient objects after the fact and you can remedy the situation, then do so. In no event should any healthcare provider proceed with any procedure without the unwavering consent of the patient. Next, never perform a procedure for the convenience of the staff. That is not a reason to violate the patient's right to refuse.

What If?
A patient needs to receive a barium swallow but refuses to swallow the contrast medium. The hospital worker in charge of the patient takes the cup and forces the patient to drink it. You are an employee and you see what has happened.

1. What are your legal and ethical responsibilities as an employee?
2. Does the patient have any rights?

Implied Consent

There are limited situations in which the courts imply consent on behalf of the plaintiff. In one of the oldest cases of implied consent, the plaintiff, an employee of the defendant, spoke no English. He was standing in line with other employees to be vaccinated. He asked no questions. He watched others being vaccinated, and when it was his turn, he held up his arm to the physician, who proceeded with the vaccination. When the plaintiff filed suit against the company and others alleging battery, the court stated the plaintiff's action clearly indicated implied consent or *implied permission* to touch him. The court dismissed the battery claim. It is highly unlikely that any similar situation would arise in medicine today, but there are circumstances when consent will be implied.

In modern medicine, consent is implied in emergency situations. The situation must be life threatening or pose a risk of significant physical injury to the patient if the procedures are not performed. Only those procedures absolutely necessary are authorized, and as soon as possible competent consent should be obtained. Only a physician can make the determination that a true emergency exists that necessitates proceeding without consent.

Ethical dilemmas can arise for healthcare professionals when treating individuals who, for religious reasons, do not allow certain procedures to be performed. If the physicians are aware of the patient's religious beliefs, then consent is not implied. If the physician is not aware, then the courts will most likely rule that consent is implied, as long as the physician had no way of knowing the religious prohibitions.

If the religious prohibitions are known, then consent is not implied, even in the case of a minor. In *Novak v. Cobb County Kennestone Hospital Authority,* the hospital obtained a court order to administer blood to a 16-year-old Jehovah's Witness. The order was entered despite the protest of the boy and his mother. Even though the mother and child brought suit after the boy had recovered, the court dismissed all claims. Without the court order, the hospital and physicians could not have proceeded with the blood transfusions. Keep in mind that a court will only order procedures in the case of a minor. If a competent adult refuses life-saving treatment, the courts will not interfere, nor will they imply consent.

To prevent allegations of battery, always have your patient's written consent to perform a procedure. Only perform the procedure authorized, and do not exceed the scope of the consent. In emergency situations, have at least two physicians certify that an emergency exists, document the certification in the patient's record, and perform only those procedures that are necessary to save a person's life or to prevent significant injury or harm. As soon as possible, obtain competent consent for the performance of additional procedures.

All states have statutes that outline when consent is implied. Healthcare providers must be aware of their individual state laws and, as advocates for the patient's rights, do all in their power to see that the law is followed.

Sexual Assault and Battery (Misconduct)

A practitioner may also face charges of battery for any sexual conduct between provider and patient, even with a patient's apparent consent. This type of battery is known as sexual assault. Such activity has been banned both by The American Psychiatric Association and by The American Medical Association's Council of Ethical and Judicial Affairs, under the guise of treatment in Opinion 8.14A (www.ama-assn.org/ama/pub/category/8503.html). The reasons for these prohibitions are clearly seen in the classic case of sexual misconduct with a patient, *DiLeo v. Nugent.* In *DiLeo,* the plaintiff was a patient of the defendant psychiatrist for several months. In an effort to work through an impasse in therapy, the psychiatrist suggested the patient undergo therapy with the use of the date-rape drug ecstasy. The patient and her psychiatrist had an "all day experimental session" with the plaintiff using ecstasy and tryptamine to boost the effect of the ecstasy. While the plaintiff was under the influence of the drug, the defendant repeatedly had sexual contact with her. In this case, the defendant was found liable not only of negligence but also of willful misrepresentation. The plaintiff was awarded $500,000. (Although the plaintiff did not sue under a theory of assault and battery, the facts of *DiLeo* clearly support those claims.)

Psychiatrists are not the only physicians who have been sued for sexual misconduct. In *Smith v. St. Paul Fire and Marine Insurance Co.,* the plaintiffs sued a family practitioner for sexually assaulting three boys he was treating for conditions totally unrelated to their sexual organs. In *St. Paul Fire and Marine Insurance Co. v. Asbury,* several women each sued a gynecologist for fondling during routine gynecological examinations. In a third

Relate to Practice

Janice is a certified medical assistant. She has been working at the Merrinton Clinic for almost 3 years and is well liked by her patients for her upbeat personality and warm demeanor. One day while talking to one of her regular patients during her assessment, the patient asks Janice if she would consider going on a date with him. He is relatively handsome and Janice has always enjoyed talking to him on his visits. How should Janice respond?

case, *St. Paul Fire and Marine Insurance Co. v. Shernow,* a dentist was sued for giving a female patient excessive doses of nitrous oxide and then sexually assaulting her. No matter what theory of liability, under no circumstances are medical practitioners, nurses, or allied health personnel to have sexual relations with their patients.

False Imprisonment

False imprisonment is the unlawful detention of a person, in which that person is deprived of personal liberty of movement against his or her will and without any authority to detain. To be falsely imprisoned, the confinement itself must be within a specific area by means of physical barriers and/or by physical force or threat of physical force, and the person must be aware of the confinement.

Legal challenges of false imprisonment generally arise in three circumstances: first, in the psychiatric setting with involuntary commitments; second, with the use of restraints, either physical or chemical; and third, in situations in which a patient attempts to leave the hospital against medical advice.

Defenses Against False Imprisonment Charges

In the psychiatric setting, the most important defense to a claim of false imprisonment is that all legal requirements for an involuntary admission are met. Requirements that must be met include the following:

1. The statutory provisions for the reason for involuntary commitment, such as danger to self or others, exist.
2. All statutory requirements for physician examination have been met in a timely manner.
3. All appropriate documentation exists in the chart to support the action of involuntary admission.
4. All the patient's rights have been followed.
5. All statutory time limits have been met, but not exceeded, for holding an individual against his or her will.

The following cases demonstrate the right and wrong ways to effect an involuntary admission.

In the case *Brand v. University Hospital,* the plaintiff was out of town when she became ill. As she was driving to the local hospital, she experienced a seizure, blacked out behind the wheel, and was involved in an accident. She was transported from the scene of the accident to the local hospital. In the emergency department, the treating physician gave her the options either of being admitted for a neurological workup or of being discharged to her home to follow up with her own neurologist. The patient chose the latter.

Because of her medical condition she called friends to drive her home. One of her coworkers, a former drug addict, assumed the patient's behavior was due to a drug problem, and she transported the patient to the behavioral treatment unit of University Hospital. The patient was so groggy she fell asleep and did not realize where she was.

The next morning when the plaintiff awoke and realized she was in a locked psychiatric ward, she asked to be transferred to a medical ward of the hospital. She requested that the physician call the other hospital and call her neurologist. Neither the physician nor the hospital staff listened to the plaintiff for more than 36 hours. The trial court originally dismissed the plaintiff's claim, but the appeals court overturned that decision and the plaintiff was allowed to proceed against the hospital staff and physician.

In this case, the statutory requirements for an involuntary admission were not met. There was no documentation that the patient was a danger to herself or others. There was insufficient physician examination. The staff of the behavioral unit had no right to detain the plaintiff without proper and timely acquisition of the appropriate release information.

In contrast, in *Mawhirt v. Ahmed,* a patient brought suit against the hospital, physicians, and nurses for false imprisonment secondary to an involuntary admission and the use of both physical and chemical restraints. The difference between this case and *Brand* is that the physicians and staff had well documented the severe psychiatric state of the patient. The plaintiff was suffering from paranoid delusions that the CIA and Mafia were trying to harm him. Two physicians determined he was a danger to himself and others and proceeded with the appropriate procedures for the involuntary admission.

The nursing staff documented the psychotic, delusional behavior of the plaintiff as well as behavior by which the plaintiff could harm himself or threaten other patients. They followed the institution's guidelines for the administration of chemical restraints and the procedures established for the use of physical restraints. As such, the court had no difficulty in dismissing the plaintiff's claims.

Documentation of the behavior necessitating the use of restraints is critical. Under no circumstances are restraints to be used for the convenience of the staff to control an unruly patient. Your institution's policy must be clear regarding the following:

1. What circumstances necessitate the use of restraints?
2. How are restraints to be used and for what length of time?
3. What type of monitoring is required of the restrained patient?
4. What documentation is adequate to justify the use of these restraints?
5. How often must the physician reorder the use of a physical restraint?

Inadequate proof of the patient's condition or need for an involuntary admission was an issue in *Davis v. St. Jude Medical Center.* The plaintiff was a patient on a medical unit for the treatment of pancreatitis. Approximately 3 weeks after this admission, a staff physician involuntarily admitted him to the hospital's chemical dependency unit. The plaintiff repeatedly requested to be released. He even put his request in writing to the hospital's administration. He brought a habeas corpus hearing but was discharged before the hearing took place. He then brought an action for *false imprisonment.* In allowing the patient to proceed with his action, the court ruled that the hospital and physicians had failed to provide the court sufficient proof (documentation) of the necessity of the patient's involuntary admission or necessity of treatment.

Use of restraints is not limited to the psychiatric setting. In many hospitals and nursing homes, patients are restrained to prevent injury. Even using side rails on a bed is a form of restraint and thus the medical reasons for raising side rails should be documented in the record. If, after that, the patient refuses to allow the side rails to be used, he or she must sign a release from liability in the event of a fall. Even though it is probably not worth the paper it is written on in a court of law, a release gives the patient the opportunity to appreciate the gravity of his or her decision to refuse the side rails. Use of any other type of restraint, such as sheets to hold patients in wheelchairs, posey belts, or any other form of physical restraint, should be implemented only as a last resort and must be used only as approved by hospital policy and the physician. In all situations, when possible obtain written consent for the use of any type of restraint.

Restraints in the Home-Care Setting

It is highly recommended that home-care personnel not place patients in restraints. Home-care personnel are not available for a sufficient amount of time to evaluate the patient's response to the restraints, to evaluate the need for continued use of restraints, to determine whether the restraints are being used properly, or to determine how the patient is being monitored while in restraints. If the family puts the patient in restraints, notify the physician, obtain an order, and instruct the family of the proper care of a patient in restraints.

Against Medical Advice

Another situation that raises possible issues of false imprisonment involves patients wishing to leave the hospital against medical advice (AMA). Although you have an obligation to review with the patient all the possible complications that could arise should he or she leave AMA, you cannot prevent a competent patient from refusing treatment or leaving. This means you cannot physically bar the patient's exit. You cannot prevent the patient from collecting clothes and other personal belongings, and you cannot attempt to touch the patient in an effort to make him or her stay.

In a particularly serious case, a 67-year-old man was physically prevented from leaving a nursing home for 51 days. Shortly after his nephew admitted him to the nursing home, the man attempted to leave. Nursing home employees forcibly returned him. The man continued to demand his release and made several additional attempts to leave the home. He was finally placed in a restraint chair and denied use of the phone or even access to his own clothes. The court found that the actions of the staff were in complete and utter disregard of the man's rights and were willful, reckless, and malicious in detaining him. When the patient is competent, he cannot be detained against his will.

If a situation exists where the patient is clearly not competent, then a hospital may be justified in detaining the patient. In *Blackman for Blackman v. Rifkin,* the patient was extremely intoxicated and had suffered head trauma. The court ruled that the hospital was justified in restraining the patient and keeping her in the hospital because the hospital could assume that the patient would have consented to treatment if she had not been in that condition. The court dismissed her false imprisonment suit. This case must be limited to its facts. Although the hospital may be justified in detaining a severely intoxicated person, the hospital cannot detain a competent patient against his or her will.

In the case of a minor, the hospital can attempt to obtain a court order to require the family to keep the child in the hospital, but any attempt to physically restrain the child or the parent in the absence of a court order exposes the hospital to liability. Basically, you can talk to a patient until he refuses to listen to you, but you cannot physically prevent him from leaving (Figure 7-2).

It does not matter how noble your motives are. Patients have a right to refuse treatment. Patients also have a right to leave the hospital when they wish (unless they have been committed through legal procedures) and to have freedom of movement. As healthcare providers, you cannot interfere with these rights without potential liability.

One other scenario may result in an action for false imprisonment. When the physician has written a discharge order, the hospital cannot keep the patient until he or she "settles the bill." Even though the patient obviously has the obligation to pay for services rendered, the hospital cannot hold the patient until the patient indicates how he or she will pay for services.

Intentional Infliction of Emotional Distress

To establish the tort of intentional infliction of emotional distress, the plaintiff must show that the defendant's conduct is outrageous and beyond the bounds of common decency. Insulting behavior is not enough; the actions must be egregious. One case in

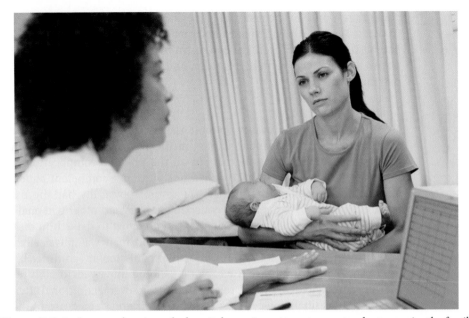

Figure 7-2 In the case of a minor, the hospital can attempt to get a court order to require the family to keep the child in the hospital, but any attempt to physically restrain the child or the parent in the absence of a court order exposes the hospital to liability.

which the court allowed the plaintiff to proceed with his claim of intentional infliction of emotional distress is *Williams v. Payne et al.* In *Williams,* the police suspected that the plaintiff had ingested crack cocaine. The plaintiff was brought to Pontiac Osteopathic Hospital, where the sheriff asked the physician to pump the plaintiff's stomach. The physician was aware that the sheriff did not have a warrant for the search.

After placing the plaintiff in four-point restraints, the physician forcefully and over the objections of the plaintiff performed a gastric lavage. Thereafter, the plaintiff was involuntarily catheterized. In refusing to dismiss the claims against the hospital and physician, the court concluded that a jury could decide whether the conduct was outrageous.

Trespass to Land

The tort of trespass to land occurs when a person, without the consent of the owner, enters on another's land or causes anyone or anything to enter the land. Harm to the land is not required, but without harm to the land, courts usually award only nominal damages. Trespass to land arises most often in the home health area.

In home care, healthcare providers are guests in the patients' homes. They are there to perform necessary medical procedures and to teach, but they are still guests in the patients' homes. At any time that a patient instructs you to leave his or her home, you must leave; if you do not leave, you commit trespass to land. Keep in mind that the landowner is authorized to use reasonable force to remove a trespasser. Even if your motives are noble in refusing to leave the property, such as wanting to perform necessary wound care for the patient's benefit, your intent is no defense to the tort of trespass. Other potential claims for trespass to land include those against the patient who refuses to leave a facility after being discharged and against visitors in a facility who refuse to leave after visiting hours.

Quasi-Intentional Torts

Quasi-intentional torts include defamation, invasion of privacy, and breach of confidentiality. *Quasi* means "resembling." These types of torts resemble intentional torts but are different because they are based on speech.

Defamation

Defamation is a false statement that wrongfully damages the reputation of another person. Libel refers to written, printed, or visual defamatory statements, and slander refers to spoken defamatory statements. To be liable for defamation, you must make a defamatory statement that is published or broadcast to third parties; you cannot defame someone by telling only the person. Finally, the speaker must know or should know that the statement is false.

In defining a defamatory statement, the courts have looked to whether the statement exposed the plaintiff to public hatred, contempt, ridicule, or degradation. There must be proof that there was actual harm to the person's reputation.

There are, however, certain statements that are considered *defamatory statements per se,* such as serious allegations of sexual misconduct or criminal behavior or allegations that the plaintiff is afflicted with a loathsome disease. Historically, loathsome diseases include syphilis, gonorrhea, and leprosy. Today, allegations of having hepatitis, being human immunodeficiency virus (HIV) positive, or being diagnosed with acquired immunodeficiency syndrome (AIDS) may well be the new loathsome diseases. In the case of *defamatory statements per se,* the plaintiff does not need to prove actual damage to reputation.

An example of a *defamation statement per se* case is *Schlesser v. Keck.* The plaintiff was a cook and caterer who tested false-positive for syphilis when she was in the army. She sought treatment for the false-positive diagnosis. The defendant was the physician's nurse, who was administering the treatments. Despite the defendant's knowledge that the tests were false-positive and the defendant's knowledge that the plaintiff did not have syphilis, the defendant announced at a party that the plaintiff had syphilis and should not be allowed to cater or prepare food.

Defenses of Defamation

Truth is an absolute defense to defamation. Even if a true statement damages a person's reputation, it is not actionable as defamation. Certain individuals, such as public officials, must prove actual malice on the part of the defendant before they are allowed to succeed.

In addition to the previously mentioned situations, there may be qualified privileges that protect a person from a defamation suit. One of the most common is the qualified privilege all states have enacted concerning the reporting of elder or child abuse. As long as the report is made in good faith, the healthcare provider is protected from liability. Most states have also granted peer review members a qualified privilege. Such individuals must be members of a properly convened peer review committee; the committee must be duly authorized by the facility to conduct peer review; and the comments made in the committee meeting and all reports of the committee must be confidential. At the same time, although the members of a peer review committee may have a qualified privilege to speak freely within the confines of the committee, that privilege does not extend to speaking freely about the committee findings or proceedings to individuals not involved with the peer review committee.

The greatest liability for defamation suits results from statements made about coworkers, especially when future employers seek references.

In *Ironside v. Simi Valley Hospital,* a physician sued the hospital for sending an unsolicited letter to the physician's new employer stating that the physician previously had his privileges summarily suspended and that a report to that effect had been sent to the California Medical Board. The letter suggested that the new employer check the status of the physician's license to practice medicine with the California Medical Board. In actuality, there had been no suspension or limitation placed on the physician's license. The letter, however, did imply that there had been. Likewise, in *Simpkins v. District of Columbia et al.,* the court held that a plaintiff physician could proceed against defendants who allegedly reported to a physician data bank that the physician had resigned his staff privileges at the hospital during a review of the quality of care he provided.

The advantage is, even though a qualified privilege exists to give a good-faith assessment of an employee's job performance, many businesses have opted only to verify dates of employment to avoid any allegation of defamation. Under no circumstances should anyone give his or her unsolicited opinion about a former employee.

Invasion of Privacy

Invasion of privacy is the tort of unjustifiably intruding upon another's right of privacy by any of the following actions:

1. Appropriating his or her name or likeness
2. Placing a person in a false light
3. Publishing private facts
4. Unreasonably interfering with his or her seclusion

Invasion of privacy differs from defamation. In most instances, the information is true but is information that a person wants to keep private. Although defamation causes injury to reputation, invasion of privacy causes injury to feelings.

Appropriating Likeness and Placing a Person in a False Light

In the medical setting the most common example of appropriating likeness is the use of photographs or video images of the patient without consent or exceeding the scope of the consent. For example, in *Vassiliades v. Garfinckel's, Brooks Brothers,* a plastic surgeon used before-and-after pictures of a patient in a public demonstration without the patient's consent. Another example is the use of a video of a cesarean section not for medical teaching purposes but for inclusion in a movie that was shown publicly in movie theaters *(Feeney v. Young).*

If a patient gives consent to the use of his or her likeness for teaching purposes or treatment purposes, the scope of the consent cannot be exceeded. If the patient does not give consent, then no likeness can be used at all for any reason.

What If?

A local politician has extensive cosmetic dental work and plastic surgery performed in the hospital and clinic where you work. You tell your family, and the patient learns of this from someone in the local community. In other words, her privacy has been breached.

What are the legal and ethical ramifications?

Publicizing Private Facts

The most basic right of patients is to expect healthcare professionals to keep all information obtained in the treatment of the patient confidential. Every state mandates that the patient's confidentiality be maintained. Every state outlines only limited situations in which a person may release information concerning a patient without his or her consent.

In *Estate of Behringer v. Princeton Medical Center,* a successful ear, nose, and throat surgeon who practiced at the medical center was admitted for tests and diagnosed with AIDS. No special steps were taken to protect the medical record or the patient's privacy. In fact, the physicians and nurses who cared for the surgeon spoke openly about his condition to individuals who had no involvement in his care. By the time the physician was discharged from the hospital, numerous persons in the community knew of his condition and his practice was adversely affected.

In holding that the physician could bring suit against the medical center for invasion of privacy, the court stated: "The information was too easily available, too titillating to disregard. All that was required was a glance at the chart, and the written words became whispers and the whispers became roars." The whispers should never have taken place.

Likewise, in *Doe v. Methodist Hospital,* the plaintiff suffered a heart attack and was taken to the hospital by paramedics. He disclosed his HIV status to the paramedics. They noted this on their report, which became part of the medical record. One of the plaintiff's coworkers called his wife, who was a nurse at the hospital, and she reviewed the patient's records and told her husband the plaintiff's HIV status. While the Indiana Supreme Court ruled that Indiana does not recognize the tort of invasion of privacy, the suit was allowed to proceed under other causes of actions.

Even disclosing information to other healthcare professionals may lead to a lawsuit. In *Saur v. Probes,* the plaintiff's wife attempted to have the plaintiff involuntarily committed for psychiatric treatment. She went to court and the court appointed a psychiatrist to examine the plaintiff. The court-appointed psychiatrist contacted the defendant, who had been the plaintiff's treating physician for several months. The two physicians discussed the plaintiff's medical condition. The plaintiff filed the action against his treating psychiatrist, alleging that the psychiatrist disclosed confidential information obtained during the course of treatment without his permission. The lower court dismissed the plaintiff's case, but the higher court reversed this decision, finding that the plaintiff was entitled to have his case heard before a jury to decide whether the disclosure was appropriate. Whether this plaintiff ultimately wins is not the issue. The issue is that the court allowed the case to proceed to the jury.

Being a healthcare provider and working in a medical facility do not give you the right to unlimited access to all patients' medical records. The law allows you to view and use only the medical records of the patients you are treating.

These cases teach some important lessons. Disclosure of confidential patient information may lead to lawsuits and disciplinary actions under legal theories of liability such as the following:

- Breach of contract
- Breach of confidentiality
- Negligence
- Intentional infliction of emotional distress
- Defamation

Breach of Confidentiality

The computer age is creating even more problems for breach of confidentiality. While allowing practitioners to have easier access to their patient records and allowing information to be relayed more quickly, computerized medical records permit too many people access. A case in point was filed in 1997 in Fulton County, Georgia. In *Ruocco v. Emory Hospital,* the plaintiff filed a lawsuit alleging invasion of privacy, negligent maintenance of records, negligent supervision, intentional infliction of emotional distress, and defamation.

The plaintiff was a nurse, employed by the hospital, who was taking part in a hepatitis study. She received injections as part of the study. When she missed several weeks of work, one of the physicians in the study accessed her electronic medical record without the plaintiff's permission. Although he was not the plaintiff's treating physician, he accessed the records by claiming he was. He did not tell the plaintiff he accessed the records and, in fact, in his deposition he stated that he never intended to tell her. The plaintiff learned of the unauthorized access when she accessed her own records and saw that someone had accessed her records without her consent.

The concern over electronic access to medical records has been increasing. In 1996, Congress enacted the *Health Insurance Portability and Accountability Act of 1996 (HIPAA),* calling for regulations to establish criteria for a federal standard in authorizing the release of medical information. In February 2000 the U.S. Department of Health and Human Services published the final rules to establish the federal criteria.

Whether a healthcare provider has access to the traditional written medical record or to computerized records, the responsibility to keep information confidential does not change (Figure 7-3). Any information that a healthcare provider learns while taking care of a patient is confidential, even if it does not relate directly to the treatment of the patient.

The issue of confidentiality is both a legal and an ethical issue. The code of ethics of allied health personnel must emphasize that the healthcare professional must safeguard the patient's right to privacy by judiciously protecting confidential information. Many other groups, such as the Hospice Association of America, the American Nurses Association, the National League for Nursing, and the American Hospital Association, recognize as a basic right of patients the confidentiality of the assessments, treatment, and information contained in the patient's medical records.

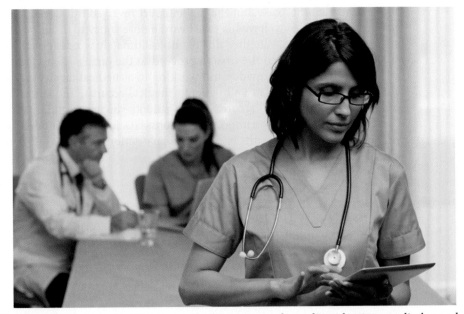

Figure 7-3 Whether a healthcare provider has access to the traditional written medical record or to computerized records, the responsibility to keep information confidential does not change.

Intentional and Quasi-Intentional Torts and Insurance Policies

Even though medical malpractice polices have historically covered intentional torts, many insurers are writing exclusions from coverage. This is especially true if the tort alleged involves sexual misconduct. As a healthcare provider, know what your policy covers and what it does not.

What If?

An adult patient is a member of a religion that does not believe in receiving blood. The patient receives a colostomy and begins hemorrhaging. He is unable to voice his objections. You know of this patient's strong beliefs and that he does not want to receive blood. On the admission sheet, the area for religion is blank. He has no family. The nurses and physicians want to give blood and you do not want him to die.

1. What should you do?
2. What are the ethical dilemmas and legal implications if he receives blood?
3. What are the legal and ethical implications if the patient is a minor and the parents refuse blood?

What If?

An Alzheimer's patient strikes you in the face and breaks your nose. You strike back to defend yourself and you injure the patient.

1. What are the ethical and legal implications?
2. Can you file a claim for workers' compensation because you received an injury while working?
3. What are the patient's rights?

Conclusion

The performance of daily patient care and treatment gives rise to potential liability for intentional and quasi-intentional torts. You can avoid liability if you always have your patient's consent to perform specific procedures and do not exceed that consent. Always maintain your patient's confidentiality and speak only to those individuals who are actively involved in the patient's care. Understand that your patient has an absolute right to refuse treatment and that your ability to change a person's mind is limited to your verbal skills only. It is not true that every patient is a potential plaintiff. However, a patient can become a plaintiff if you do not exercise good nursing judgment or do not have respect for your patient's rights, privacy, and freedom.

Chapter Review Questions

1. Publishing private but true facts about someone is defined as
   A. libel.
   B. slander.
   C. invasion of privacy.
   D. negligence.

2. If a patient has given consent for a procedure and a different or separate procedure is performed, the physician can be held liable for
   A. defamation.
   B. battery.
   C. assault.
   D. invasion of privacy.

3. Knowingly printing or publishing false information about someone is known as
   A. invasion of privacy.
   B. slander.
   C. breach of confidentiality.
   D. libel.

4. If you raise your hand or fist in such a manner that another person becomes fearful that you are going to strike him or her, you have committed
   A. assault.
   B. battery.
   C. defamation.
   D. libel.

5. A patient is scheduled to have a procedure performed, but states that he or she does not want the procedure. If the healthcare professional disregards the patient's wishes and performs the procedure anyway, the provider has just committed
   A. assault.
   B. invasion of privacy.
   C. breach of confidentiality.
   D. battery.

Self-Reflection Questions

1. How does intent play a role in an intentional tort?
2. How does consent play a role in the defense of an intentional tort?
3. How can you help ensure a patient's privacy?
4. How can charting help prevent a successful lawsuit based on false imprisonment?

Internet Activities

1. Using legal websites and search engines, find a case based on a lack of informed consent in your area.
2. Perform a web search for informed consent. What information must be disclosed during informed consent and who is responsible for obtaining the informed consent?

Bibliography

Aiken T, editor: *Legal, ethical, and political issues in nursing*, ed 2, Philadelphia, 2004, F.A. Davis.

Big Town Nursing Home, Inc. v. New, 461 S.W.2d 195 (Tex. 1970).

Blackman for Blackman v. Rifkin, 759 P.2d 54 (Colo. 1988).

Brand v. Univ. Hosp., 525 S.E.2d 374 (Ga. 1999).

Davis v. St. Jude Med. Ctr., 645 So. 2d 771 (La. App. 5th Cir. 1994).

DiLeo v. Nugent, 592 A.2d 1126 (Md. 1991).

Doe v. Methodist Hosp., 639 N.E.2d 683 (Ind. 1994, rev'd, 690 N.E.2d 681) (Ind. 1997).

Estate of Behringer v. Princeton Med. Ctr., 592 A.2d 1251 (N.J. 1991).

Id. at 1273.

Feeney v. Young, 191 A.D. 501, 181 N.Y. Supp. 481 (N.Y. 1920).

Guin v. Sison, 552 So. 2d 60 (La. 1989).

Ironside v. Simi Valley Hosp., No. 95-6336, slip op. (6th Cir. 1996).

Mawhirt v. Ahmed, 86 F.Supp.2d 81 (E.D. N.Y. 2000).

Montgomery v. Bazaz-Shegal, 742 A.2d 1125 (Pa. 1999).

Novak v. Cobb County Kennestone Hosp. Auth., No. 94-8403, slip op. (11th Cir. 1996).

O'Brien v. Cunard S.S. Co., 28 N.E. 266 (1881).

Phipps v. Clark Oil and Ref. Corp., 408 N.W. 2d 569, 573 (Minn. 1987).

Pizzaloto v. Wilson, 437 So. 2d 859 (La. 1983).

Roberson v. Provident House, 576 So. 2d 992 (La. 1991).

Ruocco v. Emory Hosp., No. 97-VS0132401.

Saur v. Probes, 476 N.W.2d 496 (Mich. 1991).

Schlesser v. Keck, 271 P.2d 588 (Calif. 1954).

Schloendorff v. Soc'y of N.Y. Hosp., 105 N.E. 92 (1914).

Simpkins v. District of Columbia et al., No. 94-5243, slip op. (D.C. Cir. 1997).

Smith v. St. Paul Fire and Marine Ins. Co., 353 N.W.2d 130 (Minn. 1984).

St. Paul Fire and Marine Ins. Co. v. Asbury, 720 P.3d 540 (Ariz. 1986).

St. Paul Fire and Marine Ins. Co. v. Shernow, 610 A.2d 1281 (Conn. 1992).

Vassiliades v. Garfinckel's, Brooks Bros., 492 A.2d 580 (D.C. 1985).

Williams v. Payne et al., 73 F. Supp. 2d 785 (E.D. Mich. 1999).

Additional Resources

www.ama.org

www.apa.org

www.ast.org

www.aama-ntl.org

www.loc.gov

Chapter 8

Statutory Reporting and Public Duties

Jeanne McTeigue

Abuse A misuse or improper use of something. In relationships, it is the pattern of misuse or inappropriate treatment systematically to gain control and power over another individual.

Addiction Habit or behavior whose compulsive draw enslaves the individual.

Child Abuse Prevention and Treatment Act of 1974 Law enacted in 1974 that requires the reporting of child abuse or suspected abuse.

Communicable disease Specific disease or illness that can cause an epidemic or pandemic to the general public.

Coroner Physician or pathologist appointed to perform autopsies and testing to determine cause of death and time of death in suspicious deaths or under circumstances when no person was in attendance of the death.

Employee assistance program (EAP) Program designed to help employees receive counseling for substance abuse or other issues of abuse, without fear of losing their jobs; may offer legal and financial counseling as well.

Inquest Investigation into a suspicious death, including autopsy and other investigation, to determine time and cause of death.

Postmortem Examination that is performed on an individual after death.

Vital statistics (public) Community-wide recording of individual key human events such as births, deaths, marriages, or divorces.

CHAPTER OBJECTIVES

1. Describe what is meant by statutory reporting duties required of healthcare professionals.
2. Explain the reasons for documentation of vital statistics.
3. Explain components of a birth or death certificate and describe when a physician or coroner needs to sign one.
4. Identify the communicable and sexually transmitted diseases that must be reported.
5. Describe child, spousal, elder, and sexual abuse and possible signs of abuse.
6. Explain the function of an employee assistance program (EAP).
7. Explain addiction and regulations of controlled substances and the DEA schedule of drugs.

Introduction

State and federal guidelines and statutes require all facilities and businesses connected to the general public to maintain standards to ensure that the public is safe. For instance, a restaurant needs to be inspected regularly for cleanliness and adherence to food storage guidelines to ensure that the general public is safe from possible diseases and illnesses. In the area of medicine and medical professional careers, there are even more guidelines and statutes. If these guidelines and standards are not met, a facility or clinic can be closed.

Those in the healthcare field must understand that they are held to the highest professional standards and that the lives and well-being of their patients and the general public must always be their utmost concern. For that reason, it is the duty of the healthcare professional to report and document incidents of concern for a patient's safety and well-being, as well as the well-being of the public at large. The healthcare professional also has a duty to maintain strict, accurate documentation of events that affect and contribute to the **vital statistics** of the public, such as births and deaths. This chapter will detail some of the general guidelines and expectations of the healthcare professional's responsibility to both their patients and the general public.

Statutory Report Duties

Statutory report duties, in the healthcare field, refer mainly to the responsibility of healthcare providers to report areas of vital information to the necessary agencies as deemed necessary for the welfare of the general public. These may vary between states, but, overall, some of the events requiring accurate documentation and (in some cases) prompt reporting include the following:

- Births
- Deaths
- Communicable diseases
- Assaults or criminal acts
- Abuse—child, elder, or spousal
- Substance abuse

Vital Statistics and Public Health Records

Statistical tracking over the centuries has long included the recording of births, deaths, reasons for deaths, and illnesses. In fact, maintaining the trends of diseases and illnesses that cause mortality (death) or morbidity (illnesses) has existed since the seventeenth century. It was this actual tracking that was initially used to create the International Classification of Diseases (ICD), or the code set that is used by healthcare providers for diagnosis of their patients. The resultant records are maintained by the Centers for Medicare and Medicaid Services (CMS) and the U.S. Department of Health and Human Services (HHS). Coding of accurate diagnoses using this coding system is mandated for all healthcare facilities and providers, and reporting of all areas of concern for the general population, such as communicable diseases, is also mandated by local health departments as well as the federally operated Centers for Disease Control and Prevention (CDC). In addition, each state's department of health also mandates the reporting of all statistical information, such as births and deaths. Although many allied healthcare workers may assist in the completion and

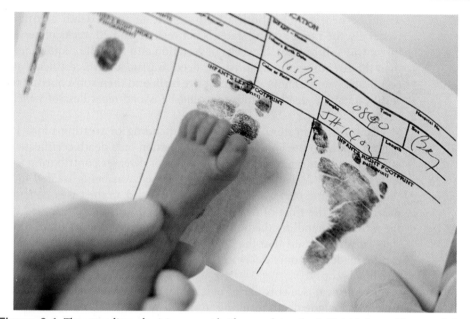

Figure 8-1 The attending physician or midwife completes the initial birth certificate and then submits it to the local (usually county) agency for recording. From there the government's official certificate of birth is released.

documentation of these events, it is ultimately the legal responsibility of the physician or provider signing the documentation to verify that the information is accurate and complete.

Births

Documentation of birth records through a valid birth certificate is the responsibility of the provider assisting with the birth. Everyone needs a valid birth certificate to acquire a Social Security number, register for school, apply for a driver's license or passport, and register to vote. For that reason, it is easy to see that the accuracy of this information is very important to each individual because it can affect so many areas of a person's life.

Generally, the information required to file for a birth certificate is the date, time, and place of the birth, as well as parental information. Once documented, a record of a live birth (Figure 8-1) is filed by the midwife or hospital (if birth occurs there) and submitted to the local (usually county) agency for recording. This must be signed by the physician or provider who assisted in the birth. This form is then taken by the local county clerk and recorded, and an official birth certificate is issued for the individual. Depending on the local requirements, the form for filing of births may be more extensive to include the health of the mother of the child and/or father if known.

As with all documentation, it is important that a birth certificate be accurate, legible, and complete when submitted to the local authorities. Some states and local authorities can implement charges against individuals for incorrectly, improperly, or falsely reporting information on birth or death certificates.

Deaths

Statutory regulations vary among states regarding requirements for death certificates. For instance, in the case of a still-born child, each state has legal requirements of the fetal age that would constitute identification as "a child," thereby determining when it would be necessary for both a birth certificate and a death certificate to be issued. Generally, the range among states is between 18 and 20 weeks of gestation. Thus, if an infant was still-born at 22 weeks of gestation and the state requirement was 20 weeks, then the attending physician would need to issue a birth certificate as well as a death certificate. If an infant is a full-term live birth and then subsequently dies, both a birth certificate and a death certificate would be issued regardless of which state the birth occurs.

Death certificates are issued by the attending or treating physician in cases of a natural death. In the United States, information on a death certificate includes the following details: cause of death and illnesses or diseases contributing to the death; time and date of death; length of time the deceased was being treated for the illness that caused the death; performance of an autopsy; and, in the case of a female, existence of pregnancy at the time of death. Once the death certificate is issued by the physician, the mortuary handling the body then files it with the county office. In light of all these steps, it is important that the death certificate is signed quickly so that arrangements can be made. The only delay in transferring the patient to the mortuary should be a pending autopsy.

In some deaths, a **coroner** or official state physician would sign the death certificate. Examples include death resulting from a criminal act (homicide); lack of an attendant at death; a patient found dead at home; accidental deaths; or suicides. If there are suspicious circumstances surrounding a death, the coroner is asked to determine whether an autopsy is needed. The coroner is an elected or state-appointed physician (usually a pathologist) who is able to perform **postmortem** examinations to determine time and cause of death. It is the coroner, at that point, who will perform the autopsy and any pathological testing indicated in order to issue the death certificate with the determined cause of death and other details. If an individual dies under suspicious circumstances, an autopsy is mandated; however, in the absence of suspicious circumstances, an autopsy is not performed without the consent or request of the surviving next of kin.

What about cases of individuals who die using in-home hospice services? In most home hospice cases, because the person expired at home, even without suspicious circumstances, a coroner is called to determine whether there were any concerning factors that might warrant an **inquest.** In many states, the only exception to this situation is when the patient is older than age 90 and there is no appearance of foul play. In most cases, the coroner would perform a postmortem examination of the scene and the individual to ensure that nothing suspicious or questionable is overlooked.

The death certificate is needed for proof of death for many reasons—for banking purposes, insurance reports, and Internal Revenue Service or Social Security notification, just to name a few. The information provided must be accurate and properly documented for the surviving family to manage the estate of the deceased and finalize the settlement of their responsibilities.

Communicable Diseases

If the general population is in danger of an epidemic or disease that could be transferred to many individuals, then it is the obligation of healthcare professionals to notify the proper authorities to prepare and hopefully avoid the dissemination of that disease or illness. It is a legal and ethical mandate that these cases are reported to the local department of health and they may also need to be reported to the Centers for Disease Control and Prevention (CDC).

Not all contagious illnesses are reported as **communicable diseases.** Specific guidelines may vary from state to state regarding the information that needs to be reported,

What If?

The cause of death is unknown for an individual found dead on his living room sofa. Neighbors have called the police, who find that the individual is an elderly man, 80 years of age, who seems to have died of natural causes.

1. Would a coroner be called?
2. Would an autopsy be performed?
3. Would the family be under investigation?

but the general standards are the same. If a communicable disease, such as tuberculosis, is diagnosed at the local hospital, the hospital will automatically contact the local health department (who will in turn notify the CDC) so that an investigation can be done to determine who else might be in danger of possible exposure and to arrange for testing and treatment of those individuals, quarantining if necessary to avoid the widespread exposure of the disease.

In cases of communicable diseases, such as those listed next, there is no requirement for a HIPAA release from the patient before the authorities are notified.

The HIPAA requirement is waived in the following cases:

1. Communicable diseases
2. Criminal acts (such as rape, gunshot wounds, or stab wounds)
3. Subpoena or court order
4. Workers' compensation injuries

Although in these cases a release is not required to convey the necessary information to the necessary parties, this does not in any way allow for the arbitrary release of information, only for the release of details to the necessary authorities or agencies that need to be informed.

All states will vary in their list of required reportable illness/diseases, but the following diseases are generally standard ones that would need to be reported:

- Tuberculosis
- Rubeola
- Rubella
- Tetanus
- Diphtheria
- Cholera
- Rheumatic fever
- Poliomyelitis (polio)
- Acquired immunodeficiency syndrome (AIDS)
- Meningitis
- Certain strands of influenza (such as swine flu)
- Sexually transmitted diseases

In most cases, the local health department would be called if time were of the essence, but some reports can just be filed by mail to the health department, who would then investigate and follow up as needed. The reporting provider would have to submit the name, address, and occupation of the individual involved; the disease or suspected disease involved; and the date of onset of that disease, submitting all this with his or her own credentials and information.

Childhood vaccinations have provided us with immunizations from many of these diseases listed, and most schools require up-to-date immunizations for enrollment. These measures have gone a long way in preventing many of these diseases from becoming current health hazards, but cases do still exist. Other diseases that often need to be reported are rabies; pertussis (whooping cough); hepatitis A, B, or C; measles, mumps, or rubella; and tetanus. Again, although most people are immunized from these diseases, cases do still exist, and the potential for the spread of these diseases, therefore, is still a danger.

Most area health departments also require that injuries such as dog bites or other animal encounters as well as illnesses acquired from public places or businesses be reported so they are able to track and record any possible problems or incidents that endanger the public.

Discussion

A patient is seen in the emergency department because of a severe cough and he is expectorating blood. What steps should be taken by the providers in the emergency department?

Sexually Transmitted Diseases/AIDS

Sexually transmitted diseases are reportable to the local health departments, either by phone or via mail. If a provider notifies a patient that he or she has a sexually transmitted disease, the provider must also counsel the patient regarding the risks and contagious nature of that specific disease and encourage the patient to have any partners tested and treated accordingly.

In the case of human immunodeficiency virus (HIV) and the manifestation of that virus, which is acquired immunodeficiency syndrome (AIDS), again the provider must counsel the patient regarding exposure and partners who might also be at risk. The health department would also be notified and would follow up with the patient regarding others who might be at risk as well. In each state there are specific requirements regarding patients and healthcare workers reporting positive cases. Rules vary among states regarding whether the provider or the laboratory is required to report the cases. Most states require any cases be reported within 30 days of diagnosis, while some states permit only 10 days to report positive cases.

A patient may be HIV positive and not have AIDS. A provider is bound both legally and ethically to treat a patient who has this disease. Providers may not refuse to treat any patient who has a positive diagnosis. The usual and proper precautions for any blood-borne pathogen should be followed to protect the healthcare providers who are treating the patient.

Laws regarding the reporting of HIV/AIDS vary, but many of the states have statutes that enable the provider or the local health departments to contact any known partners, spouses, or needle-sharing companions, for example, of exposure to the virus. Again, the provider or health department should counsel the patient on the moral obligation to notify anyone who would possibly be at risk of contracting the virus. The patient should also be counseled that in some states criminal charges can be filed against anyone who knowingly exposes another person to the virus without the partner being aware of the risk.

Discussion
A patient known to be HIV positive has an appointment at your office. Several of the workers are hesitant to assist the physician during this patient's exams. Does the medical assistant have the right to refuse to assist the physician with a patient who is known as an HIV-positive patient?

HIV/AIDS and the Healthcare Worker

Years ago, when the HIV virus was still an unknown disease, many patients were exposed from blood transfusions and other types of exposure made during diagnostic or therapeutic procedures. Since then, many screening processes have been initiated to ensure the safety of any blood or other donor candidates from possible communicable diseases. Because AIDS is a fatal disease, it is extremely important to eliminate all risks of exposure.

Anyone working in a high-risk area should receive routine screenings from their employer, and follow-up care if exposed. If a worker has a needle stick exposure, the OSHA guidelines indicate that the exposed worker is screened immediately (at the cost of the employer) and then offered treatment and follow-up screening 6 months after the exposure. This should be initiated within 2 hours of the exposure. Furthermore, OSHA guidelines also require the employer to ask the patient the source of the needle or sharps, so that if other individuals are at risk they can be offered the opportunity to be tested at the same time. However, most states do not require the mandatory testing of the patient, nor can the provider affected test that patient's blood without the patient's consent.

Healthcare workers who are HIV positive are not required, at this time, to disclose their HIV status to their patients. There is little risk for patients to be exposed by providers, and therefore it is believed that the privacy of the provider should be protected. However, if universal precautions are not employed by a provider who is HIV positive or instruments are not properly sterilized, then the risk for exposure is increased. There are a couple of cases concerning two dentists, one in Oklahoma and another in Florida, who were charged with exposing patients. The Florida case claimed that five patients were exposed to HIV from the dentist himself, who was HIV positive. In the Oklahoma case, the dentist was reusing needles and not following OSHA guidelines for sterilization and universal precautions. As a result, more than 7000 patients were at risk and were thus offered screenings for HIV and hepatitis; the dentist had his license suspended and was facing charges. The Florida case is discussed in more detail in the following Discussion box.

Abuse

Abuse is defined as the misuse of something. In regard to relationships, abuse goes much farther and involves inflicting deliberate emotional, physical, psychological, and/or sexual trauma on another individual to satisfy a desire to control and have power over others. An abusive person uses physical force, mental degradation, intimidation, and other manipulative means to gain power over another individual. Specific forms that abuse can take include the following actions:

- *Physical*—pushing, hitting, shoving and punching, biting or choking, physically trapping or impeding movement

Discussion

CASE STUDY—KIMBERLY ANN BERGALIS

Bergalis was one of six patients infected with HIV after visiting David J. Acer, the Florida dentist who had AIDS. This incident is the first known case of clinical transmission of HIV. See www.nytimes.com/1991/12/09/obituaries/kimberly-bergalis-is-dead-at-23-symbol-of-debate-over-aids-tests.html.

The claim asserted that Dr. Acer infected others with HIV and that his patients were unaware of his status. As a result, one of those patients, Kimberly Ann Bergalis, died of AIDS at the age of 23. In addition to being the first known clinical transmission, it also bears the designation as being the first known case of a transmission of the disease that was "innocent exposure" during a dental procedure. Investigation into this case, in the 1980s, proved that Dr. Acer was not using universal precautions—he was working on patients without any gloves and reusing unsterilized instruments. As a result of this case, in 1985 OSHA began to require that all healthcare providers use universal precautions when treating any patients in any area of healthcare.

1. Should it be mandated that healthcare workers with a positive HIV status must inform their patients?
2. What can be done, specifically, to prevent exposures?
3. What consequences should be facing a provider who takes these actions today?

From Lambert B: Kimberly Bergalis is dead at 23; symbol of debate over AIDS tests, *The New York Times,* Dec 9, 1991, accessed at www.nytimes.com/1991/12/09/obituaries/kimberly-bergalis-is-dead-at-23-symbol-of-debate-over-aids-tests.html; Ciesielski CA, Marianos DW, Schochetman G, Witte JJ, Jaffe HW, Division of HIV/AIDS, Centers for Disease Control and Prevention: *Ann Intern Med* 121(11):886-888, 1994; *The 1990 Florida dental investigation: the press and the science,* accessed at www.ncbi.nlm.nih.gov/pubmed/7978703.

- *Verbal/emotional*—criticizing, degrading, swearing, blaming; attacks that harm self-esteem
- *Psychological*—throwing things, punching walls, breaking things, stalking, invading privacy or space, sabotaging plans or efforts of others—all to create a sense of fear
- *Sexual*—sexual acts performed without the consent of the other or under intimidating circumstances

This is just a sampling of abusive behaviors. Statutes in each state provide more specific details describing the behaviors that are considered grounds for abuse or neglect and the penalties and proof needed to sustain the cases.

Identifying Victims of Abuse

Not all abuse victims feel safe identifying themselves as victims, but some signs of abuse anyone can look for include the following:

- Repeated injuries or bruises
- Malnutrition or signs of poor nutrition
- Unusual marks, scars, or rashes
- Bite marks
- Swelling or pain anywhere on the body, including the genital area
- Venereal disease and genital abrasions or injuries
- Unexplained fractures

- Repeated accidental injuries
- Black eyes or wearing dark glasses
- Makeup worn to hide bruising

In many cases, if an abuse victim is brought to the physician or hospital for care, the abuser is usually very nearby to ensure the patient's silence; the abuser may even speak for the patient and not allow the patient to talk. In light of this behavior, current examination standards have been initiated asserting that all patients in suspicious circumstances should be asked (while alone) whether they feel that they are "safe," and if there is any possibility that they are not safe and need assistance. This gives the patient an opportunity to gain help from the providers, because many of them are very fearful of their abusers.

Child Abuse

The **Child Abuse Prevention and Treatment Act of 1974** initiated standards that now require the reporting of all child abuse cases. All states now have similar abuse prevention mandates. Authorities must be notified of any suspected case of abuse, and a thorough investigation must be done to ensure the safety of the child and further validate, or carefully dismiss, the claim. Anyone in the healthcare profession is required to report incidents, or suspicion, of abuse to the appropriate authorities (Figure 8-2). Although no one, of course, wants to cause stress and embarrassment to innocent parties, especially good parents whose situation is misinterpreted, it is nevertheless better to report it for investigation. If a genuine suspicion is indicated and there is a probable cause for concern, then to ignore the implications may endanger the child further.

All persons involved with a child are allowed to file a complaint if abuse is suspected. This includes teachers, neighbors, or friends of the family. Most states require a verbal report of an incident, which is then immediately followed up by a written report. In most states, a confidential report can be filed and/or even anonymously filed so that there is no fear of liability or repercussions from filing a report. On the contrary, there have been cases in which physicians were held legally responsible for further abuse and injuries sustained by children when they did not report the cases to the authorities when "battered child syndrome" was suspected (e.g., *Landeros v. Flood,* 551 P.22d [Calif. 1976]).

In rarer cases of child abuse, a parent or caregiver may suffer from a psychological disorder known as *Munchausen's disease by proxy,* in which the caregiver gains attention and thrives on the attention that is achieved by making his or her children sick to gain attention from the medical professionals and family and friends, and some cases of Munchausen's disease by proxy have resulted in a child's death.

A diagnosis of *battered child syndrome* refers to a syndrome in which the child has repeated injuries or illnesses that are unexplained. As with other cases of suspected abuse, in the case of a child exhibiting these repeated symptoms, the healthcare provider must initiate a report and investigation immediately. In the case of an emergency department professional, extreme cases may involve calling authorities immediately and not allowing the parent or guardian to take the child from the hospital in order to keep the child safe.

Elder Abuse

The Older Americans Act of 1987 was designed to protect adults older than age 60 from abuse, neglect, abandonment, and exploitation; the Act made it a reportable

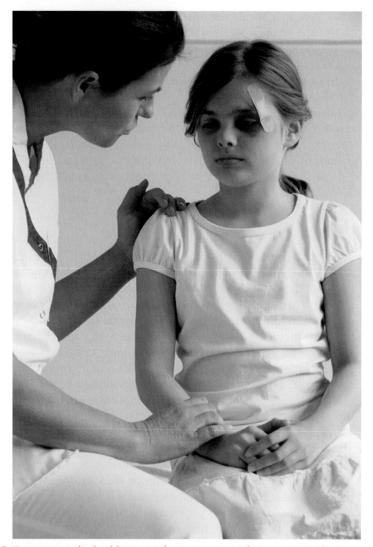

Figure 8-2 Everyone in the healthcare profession is required to report incidents, or suspicion, of child abuse to the appropriate authorities. In addition, as with other cases, the child should be asked—while alone—whether he or she feels safe.

offense in most states. The goal of this legislation is to protect the elderly in circumstances in which they are dependent on and under the care of others, such as family members participating in home care or handling the older adult's finances or other matters, as well as protecting patients in nursing homes and other facilities. In most states elder abuse is a specific criminal offense, and there are documented cases in which healthcare workers and family members alike have been charged and found guilty of elder abuse.

As in child abuse, a report may be filed without fear of civil or criminal liability, and it is the legal and ethical responsibility of all providers and healthcare workers to report any instances of suspected abuse. Also, as with child abuse, anyone can file a complaint, including friends, neighbors, other visitors to the home, or observers in public. Depending on the extent and severity of the abuse, a complaint may just be filed to establish a precedent, or, if necessary, the patient may be removed from the suspected abusive environment. For example, if a patient presented in the emergency department (ED) with trauma that was a result of an abusive situation, the emergency department would immediately report it and if necessary admit the patient until his or her safety could be secured. Again, an investigation would take place, and if appropriate, criminal charges could be filed.

The second aspect of the Older Americans Act protects elderly citizens from exploitation financially, and this is also considered a crime in the majority of states.

Relate to Practice

A patient is brought into the emergency department by her son. She is suffering from Alzheimer's dementia and is not oriented to her surroundings or family. Her son gives a history that indicates his mother fell down the stairs, but when she is examined, physical clues reveal a number of older bruises on her body, and she also exhibits a general apprehension and apparent fear of any of the male staff speaking to her or touching her.

What should be done to establish whether or not this is a true case of abuse? In addition, what evidence should be gathered in this case?

Spousal or Partner Abuse

Spousal or partner abuse is usually more complicated in terms of relationship dynamics. Spousal or partner abuse tends to cycle in frequency, often escalating in severity over time, and it will not stop without intervention. It can be frustrating for police, who want to be helpful, but partners are more difficult to permanently protect, and it typically involves a number of false starts before the abused partner is truly willing to make a permanent break from the abuser. Instead, the process of removing the victim may involve a series of events involving restraining orders or orders of protection until the patient finally realizes that more significant changes are needed.

Because of the potential for frustration connected to this cycle, police may become discouraged in responding, and allied healthcare providers familiar with the case can also experience similar burnout. Nevertheless, they are still required to report instances of observed abuse and/or suspected abuse. Again, it is important to ask questions of the patient when he or she is alone (e.g., in the emergency department) to determine whether the patient feels safe or fears for his or her safety, for example. The provider should observe the demeanor of the patient (acting apprehensive or the body language of intimidation) and should be mindful of overexaggerated concern exhibited on the part of the partner, or a partner or spouse who insists on speaking for the patient and is resistant to leaving the patient alone at all. Always attempt in these situations to speak with the patient privately to assess the situation, and it is advisable to have someone else present as a witness as well.

Sexual Assault and Abuse

Rape or sexual assault is a criminal act of violence, and as with other cases of violence, it is mandatory that the healthcare provider report the offense immediately. Police and other authorities should be immediately contacted to take the victim's statement and file a report, launching an investigation immediately. Physical examination is crucial. If a rape victim is seen in the emergency department or in any other healthcare facility, the gathering of physical evidence is extremely important to aid in prosecution of a criminal case. In any criminal case, the "chain of custody" of the evidence and the thorough gathering of evidence are vitally important; follow your state's guidelines for evidence preservation procedures.

For all cases of criminal abuse or criminal violent acts, the evidence processing might include some or all of the following:

- Photos of all injuries sustained
- Samples of urine, body fluids, specimens, or blood
- Clothing worn
- Any foreign objects involved in the crime

Finally, it is considered sexual harassment to intimidate, manipulate, or embarrass an individual in a sexual manner. Sexual harassment in the workplace has become an offense that can lead to charges and/or termination from employment. Even if an individual relays a "joke" of a sexual nature and a third party overhears the joke and feels uncomfortable or is bothered by the "joke," the individual who told the joke can face sexual harassment charges or corrective action from the employer.

Substance Abuse

Addiction is a compulsive behavior that enslaves the person to the habit, behavior, or substance to which the person is addicted. If a healthcare provider suspects, or detects, evidence of substance abuse during examination of a patient, this must be immediately reported to the proper authorities. In the instance of illegal substances, law enforcement agencies should be notified.

Keep in mind, however, that substance abuse can take place using prescription medications. For example, a patient who becomes dependent on a prescription drug may visit several different physicians to obtain an oversupply of that drug. Many go to emergency departments to try to get prescriptions or injections of that same drug. As with the other kinds of abuse discussed in this chapter, anyone can intervene to help people with addictions, and locally there are many agencies and community service departments that can be accessed to aid individuals in obtaining treatment. Many employers also have employee assistance programs (EAPs) that will also give the patients resources to help them overcome their addictions. As a healthcare provider, in addition to reporting suspected abuse, you should try to counsel the patient and recommend professional counseling to assist the patient with his or her addiction.

The Drug Enforcement Agency (DEA) and the Food and Drug Administration (FDA) oversee all providers that are licensed to prescribe drugs. Depending on the type of drug and its potential for addiction, it is limited in how much and how often prescriptions can be written and filled. The good news is that with the expansion of the electronic health record and electronic pharmacy records, it is becoming much more difficult for a person to get illegal or multiple prescriptions filled.

Until all prescriptions are electronic, however, the DEA enforces strict protocols for prescribing and distribution that include requiring certain prescriptions to be written with a triplicate copy prescription pad that is submitted to the authorities to monitor and track. The registered DEA number of the provider must appear on the prescription copy. Other categories of drugs require a written prescription and cannot be phoned or transmitted electronically to the pharmacy. In both these categories, refills are not allowed or are strictly limited. These measures were instituted to help regulate the availability of certain addictive medications and also to monitor the providers. If a healthcare provider is writing excessive prescriptions for certain medications, this process can alert authorities to the possibility of a problem with that provider.

Table 8-1 shows the DEA's classification of controlled substances. The Controlled Substances Act divides these drugs into five classes, or "schedules," with Schedule I drugs having the highest potential for abuse or addiction and Schedule V drugs having the lowest potential for abuse or addiction. Since the passing of this Act in 1970, the Act has been amended several times. Table 8-2 shows these updates.

TABLE 8-1
Drug Classifications According to the Controlled Substances Act of 1970

Drug Schedule	Characteristics	Prescription Regulations	Examples
Schedule I	High potential for abuse, severe physical or psychological dependence For research use only	No accepted use in United States Marijuana may be used for cancer and glaucoma research and may be obtained for patients in research situations	Narcotics: heroin Hallucinogens: peyote mescaline, PCP, hashish, amphetamine variants, LSD, cannabis (marijuana, THC) Designer drugs: ecstasy, crack, crystal meth
Schedule II	High potential for abuse, severe physical or psychological dependence Accepted medicinal use with specific restrictions	Dispensed by prescription only Oral emergency orders for Schedule II drugs may be given, but physician must supply written prescription within 72 hours Refills require new written prescription from physician	Narcotics: opium, codeine, morphine, methadone, hydromorphone (Dilaudid), meperidine (Demerol), oxycodone (OxyContin), fentanyl (Duragesic), pentobarbital (Nembutal) Stimulants: amphetamines, amphetamine salts (Adderall), methylphenidate (Ritalin) Depressants: pentobarbital (Nembutal)
Schedule III	Moderate potential for abuse, high psychological dependence, low physical dependence Accepted medicinal uses	Dispensed by prescription only May be refilled five times in 6 months with prescription authorization by physician Prescription may be phoned to pharmacy	Narcotics: paregoric (opium derivative), certain codeine combinations (with acetaminophen) Depressants: pentobarbital (Nembutal) (rectal route) Stimulants: benzphetamine (Didrex)
Schedule IV	Lower potential for abuse than Schedule III drugs Limited psychological and physical dependence Accepted medicinal uses	Dispensed by prescription only May be refilled five times in 6 months with physician authorization Prescription may be phoned to pharmacy	Narcotics: pentazocine (Talwin) Depressants: chloral hydrate (Noctec), phenobarbital, diazepam (Valium), chlordiazepoxide (Librium), alprazolam (Xanax), clorazepate (Tranxene), benzodiazepines (lorazepam [Ativan], flurazepam [Dalmane]), midazolam (Versed), meprobamate (Equanil), temazepam (Restoril) Stimulants: phentermine (Adipex-P)

Continued

TABLE 8-1
Drug Classifications According to the Controlled Substances Act of 1970, cont'd

Drug Schedule	Characteristics	Prescription Regulations	Examples
Schedule V	Low potential for abuse Abuse may lead to limited physical or psychological dependence Accepted medicinal uses	OTC narcotic drugs may be sold by registered pharmacist depending on state laws Buyer must be 18 years of age, show identification, and sign for medications	Preparations containing limited quantities of narcotics, generally cough and antidiarrheal preparations: cough syrups with codeine, diphenoxylate hydrochloride with atropine sulfate (Lomotil) and attapulgite (Parepectolin)

From Drug Enforcement Administration (DEA), U.S. Department of Justice, Washington, DC. Local DEA offices can provide current lists of medications on these schedules.

LSD, Lysergic acid diethylamide; *OTC,* over the counter; *PCP,* phencyclidine hydrochloride; *THC,* tetrahydrocannabinol.

TABLE 8-2
Amendments to the Controlled Substances Act of 1970

Amendment	Effect
Psychotropic Substances Act of 1978	Enabled federal government to add substances under schedules of controlled substances to the Convention of Controlled Substances (UN treaty designed to control illegal trade in psychoactive substances)
Controlled Substances Penalties Amendments Act of 1984	Strengthened penalties and removed ambiguity for both state and foreign drug felony convictions, particularly for recidivists; doubled penalties for distribution of controlled substances within 1000 feet of school property
Chemical Diversion and Trafficking Act of 1988	Implemented new provisions required by *United Nations Convention Against Illicit Traffic in Narcotic Drugs and Psychotropic Substances of 1988;* regulated chemicals and drug manufacturing equipment (effectively diminished U.S. criminal export of raw materials to cocaine manufacturers in South America)
Domestic Chemical Diversion and Control Act of 1993	Initiated registration of distributors of single-entity ephedrine products (a methamphetamine precursor); enabled DEA to revoke a company's registration without proof of criminal intent
Federal Analog Act	Enabled DEA to treat any substance intended for human consumption that is "substantially similar" to an illegal drug as if it was a Schedule I drug; designed to combat "designer drugs"

Conclusion

Public health and safety is the paramount concern of all healthcare and allied health professionals. Documentation and reporting duties must be obeyed by anyone in the medical field. It is not only a legal mandate but also, and perhaps more importantly, an ethical standard to uphold.

Chapter Review Questions

1. The acronym DEA means
   A. Drug and Ethics Administration.
   B. Drug Enforcement Agency.
   C. Drug Evaluation Agency.
   D. Drug Ethical Administration.

2. Which of the following would NOT be a possible sign of abuse?
   A. Black eyes
   B. Repeated fractures
   C. Chickenpox
   D. Unusual bruises

3. A coroner has to sign the death certificate in cases of
   A. suicides.
   B. homicides.
   C. individuals found dead in their homes younger than age 90.
   D. All of the above

4. An example of a vital statistic would be
   A. death certificates.
   B. divorce records.
   C. birth records.
   D. All the above

5. EAP means
   A. Employer assistance program
   B. Employee assistance program
   C. Equal assistance program
   D. Employee aid program

6. A characteristic that might be observed in an abused patient could be
   A. poor eye contact.
   B. guarding or guarded behavior.
   C. wearing sunglasses or makeup to hide bruises.
   D. All the above

Self-Reflection Questions
1. If you suspected a neighbor of child abuse or neglect, how would you respond?
2. What do you think would be the most difficult type of abuse to prosecute?
3. What types of evidence would you find in a criminal case of elder abuse?
4. What types of epidemics are the hardest to prevent? How can they be identified?

Internet Activities

1. Determine the laws in your state for reporting HIV/AIDS by accessing the CDC website: www.cdc.gov.
2. Read the article posted on the following website: www.ncbi.nlm.nih.gov/pmc/articles/PMC1403376/pdf/pubhealthrep00067-0011.pdf. It describes the investigation into the case of the dentist in Florida who was HIV positive. What recommendations for prevention would be most important, and what is the reality of the risk for patients now to be exposed from a healthcare provider who is HIV positive?

Additional Resources

http://emedicine.medscape.com/article/805727-treatment
www.aidshealth.org
www.cdc.gov/hiv/law/states
www.cms.gov
www.nytimes.com/1991/12/09/obituaries/kimberly-bergalis-is-dead-at-23-symbol-of-debate-over-aids-tests.html

Chapter 9

Professional Liability Insurance

Christopher Lee

KEY TERMS

Aggregate limit The maximum dollar amount your insurer will pay in total to settle your claims over the entire period of coverage.

Claims-made policy Insurance policy in which coverage is triggered on the date that the insured first becomes aware of the possibility of a claim and notifies the insurer. Commonly used with professional liability insurance such as medical and legal malpractice insurance.

Declarations page Portion of a liability insurance policy that provides basic information including the name and address of the insurance agency and agent as well as contact information for the insured individual. It also states what is insured, for how much, and under what circumstances, as well as the length of time the policy is in effect.

Disciplinary defense insurance A type of professional liability insurance that pays legal fees for the defense of the insured during disciplinary proceedings; usually included as a feature in most professional liability policies.

Excess coverage Insurance coverage that is in excess of one or more primary policies and does not pay a claim until the loss amount exceeds a specified amount. If a claim is covered by more than one policy, the second policy is said to be excess.

Exclusions A provision within an insurance policy that eliminates coverage for certain acts, types of damage, or locations.

Indemnification To compensate for loss or damage; to provide financial reimbursement to an individual in case of a specified loss.

Independent contractor A person, business, or corporation that provides goods or services to another under the terms specified in a contract or within a verbal agreement, rather than as an employee.

Insuring agreement or clause The portion of an insurance policy in which the insurer promises to make payment to or on behalf of the insured. Insuring agreements often outline a broad scope of coverage, which is then narrowed by exclusions and definitions.

Occurrence basis policy An insurance policy that covers claims taking place during the policy period, regardless of when claims are made.

Policy jacket Binder or folder containing an insurance policy; in many instances, it lists provisions common to several types of policies.

Premium The amount of money an insurer charges to provide the coverage described in the policy.

Prior acts coverage Insurance coverage for incidents that occur before the start of the policy but whose claims are made during the policy period.

Respondeat superior Legal doctrine that states in many circumstances an employer is responsible for the actions of employees performed within the course of their employment.

Self-insure A system in which a business sets aside an amount of money to provide for any losses that occur—losses that would ordinarily be covered under an insurance program. The monies that would typically be used for premium payments are added to this special fund for payment of losses incurred.

Tail coverage A provision of a claims-made liability policy that allows the insured to purchase coverage for claims made during a specified time period after the end of the policy. It covers the claim as long as the incident occurred during the time the policy was in effect.

Umbrella policy Liability insurance policy that provides protection against claims that are not covered, or are in excess of the amount covered, under a basic liability insurance policy.

Vicarious liability The liability of an employer for the actions of its designated agents. Vicarious liability can result from the acts of independent agents, partners, independent contractors, and employees.

CHAPTER OBJECTIVES

1. Define the basic liability insurance terms, concepts, and types of policies.
2. Discuss the necessity for professional liability insurance for employed health professionals and independent contractors.
3. Discuss the employer's liability policy exclusions and their effect on individual employee liability.
4. Explain the key features of a private liability policy.
5. Discuss what is covered in a disciplinary defense insurance policy.
6. List several types of private liability policies.
7. Outline the typical components of a professional liability policy.

Liability Insurance

As we have seen from previous chapters, lawsuits and litigation are a fact of life in the healthcare field. For that reason, liability insurance is also a necessary reality. The overall purpose of liability insurance is to spread the risk of financial loss among members of a group who have a commonly shared risk. A small fee, or **premium**, is paid by each insured member and put into a fund by the insurer. The insurer then uses this fund to pay for claims against any of the members. This avoids potentially devastating financial costs associated with defending yourself against such claims. Unfortunately, being innocent, even proven innocent, is no protection because even claims that have no merit can be just as costly to defend as those that do have merit. Individually, the primary objective of liability insurance is to protect your assets in the event of a judgment or settlement in favor of the claimant.

Is Your Employer's Liability Insurance All You Need?

There are two mistakes medical professionals most frequently make in believing they do not need liability insurance. First, many medical professionals believe they are adequately covered by their employers' insurance, especially because all employees pay into it. Or in some cases, employers tell employees that having their own insurance makes them targets and more likely to be sued. However, there are a host of reasons why the prudent employed professional should obtain individual professional liability insurance. The primary reason is that the employer's policy will only cover you in limited circumstances, and your interests are never of primary concern. *Instead, an employer's liability insurance is there primarily to protect the employer—not you. This is always true.* The employer's policy does not provide coverage for certain acts of the employee.

Here is an example. Suppose a medical assistant makes a remark to a coworker about a patient, and the patient overhears and perceives the remark to be defamatory. The employer's policy will probably not provide coverage for this incident, and the employee will have to defend against a lawsuit on his or her own. Even if the employee successfully defends against such allegations, the costs of doing so can be substantial. Policies are available to individuals that provide coverage for many acts that are not covered under an employer's policy.

A second reason some professionals do not see a need to obtain liability insurance is that they believe that since they do not have a lot of money, they do not have that much to protect. They believe that because they own very few assets, even if a claim against them is successful, they have little that the claimant could collect. This is a mistaken assumption. First, although a person has few assets now, it is reasonable to assume that most professionals may have assets worth protecting in the future. If a claimant secures a judgment against you, that judgment will stand and can be enforced at a later time, when your assets may have increased substantially. Purchasing insurance at that time will not help, because any prior judgments or claims will not be covered by a new policy. Besides losing a substantial portion of your assets, then, there may also be worse possibilities, such as bankruptcy.

Independent Contractors

A healthcare professional who is an independent contractor most definitely should obtain liability insurance. An independent contractor is a person who is self-employed and who enters into contracts to provide professional services to various entities such as medical facilities, physicians' offices, and/or individual clients. In general, these entities have no liability for the acts or omissions of an independent contractor unless the entity can be found directly liable, as discussed in the next section. Most of these contracting entities will require that the independent contractor show evidence of current liability coverage. Even if it is not required, securing coverage to protect your assets is exceedingly important.

Employers' Liability Policies

Of course, employees do have some coverage under their employer's liability policy— but it is not enough, and as we shall see, it may sometimes even be used against you in a case.

Let us begin, then, by having a look at what an employer's own liability policy really offers you, and how it can potentially harm your interests. An employer such as a hospital or clinic obtains professional liability insurance to protect its own interests. With respect to its liability for the negligent acts of an employee or independent contractor, the employer seeks to protect itself first against claims that fall generally under two theories of liability.

First, a claim filed may charge that the clinic or hospital itself is directly liable for the injury caused by an employee or independent contractor. Under this theory, the claimant commonly alleges one or more of the following:

1. When hiring the employee, the employer failed its duty to ascertain that the employee had the necessary qualifications and capability to render safe care.
2. The employer failed to perform a background check.
3. The employer failed to adequately supervise the employee.
4. The employer failed to provide the employee with the proper training required to render safe care or failed to properly assess that the employee required additional training.

Second, the employer can also be sued under a theory of vicarious liability, in which the acts or omissions of the employee are assigned to the employer, so that the employer can be found liable for them, invoking the legal theory called *respondeat superior,* in which the supervisor or employer is deemed responsible for the errors or actions of an employee.

Limits of Policy Exceeded

An employer's policy, as with any insurance policy, sets limits on how much the insurer pays. If an incident involves multiple alleged acts of negligence and/or claimants, it is possible that the employer's policy limits are exceeded. In that case, the employer is covered first, and the employee may be left responsible for financing all or part of the defense.

Mergers and Closures

In today's healthcare environment, the increasing number and frequency of mergers and acquisitions have resulted in complex restructuring schemes. The terms of agreement between two merging entities can result in changes in the employer's liability insurance coverage. Depending on the terms of the employer's policy and the date of an incident involving the employees, employees may find they are without employer coverage for a given incident that was covered under their employer's policy before the merger. A worse scenario can occur when a facility closes. The employer may not have purchased a policy to cover claims made after the closure, and the employee may therefore be left "bare," meaning that the insurance company will not pay for defense costs or money awards.

Conflicts Over Liability

In any given incident that results in a claim, the employer may not agree with the employee's view of that incident. For example, the employer takes the position that in a given incident the employee was not acting within the scope of his or her duties. If the employer proves this is true, the employer's insurer (or especially the employer if self-insured) has no duty to assist in the employee's defense. At the very least, the fact that the employee and the employer may disagree about the facts of an incident can create problems in the defense strategy of the insurer's attorney (Figure 9-1). It is far better to have your own policy and your own attorney whose loyalty will be only to you, the employee.

Conflicts Over Proposed Settlements

The employer may wish to settle a claim rather than defend a lawsuit for any number of reasons; for example, the employer may wish to limit negative publicity or may not want to devote the resources necessary to defend the case. The employer's insurer may settle

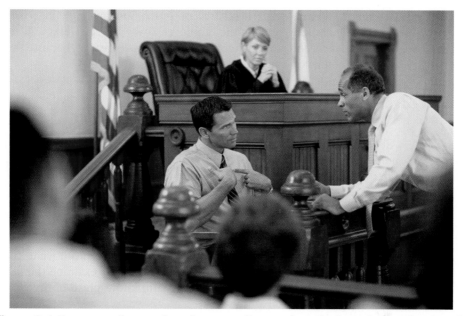

Figure 9-1 Because employee and employer may disagree about the facts of an incident, it is far better to have your own policy and your own attorney, whose loyalty will be only to you, the employee.

the claim if the claimant appears to have at least a 50% chance of winning at trial. It may be more cost-effective for the insurer to settle the case rather than risk going to trial and have a judge or jury award a substantially higher amount. Even though an employee may have strong feelings about the lack of negligence on his or her part in an incident, the best interests of the employee are not primary; those of the employer are. Once again, the insurer's loyalty is with the employer.

Conflicts Between Multiple Employees Over an Incident

Many incidents involve multiple employees. In such situations, the claimant typically sues everyone connected with the incident: the employer, the supervisors, and the employees. The potential for disagreement regarding essential facts of an incident can put an individual at odds not only with supervisors but also with coworkers, who, after all, are trying to protect themselves. Your own insurer and attorney have loyalty only to you and will formulate a defense strategy that is in your best interest rather than one that must take into account the positions of all your coworkers.

Employers' Self-Insurance

A final concern for the individual employee occurs if the employer elects to self-insure in accordance with state laws. No insurance policy is required, but an employer must provide evidence that it has sufficient funds set aside to satisfy a successful claim.

Discussion
Should all healthcare providers be required to purchase their own liability insurance? Why or why not?

Whether the employer self-insures or purchases coverage, keep in mind that the employer is looking out for the employer's own interests first and foremost. This is particularly true, however, where the employer self-insures, because then the employer has more control in the defense of a claim.

Professional Liability Insurance

All of the shortcomings just discussed help to highlight the inherent risks in relying on an employer's liability policy to protect you. The upshot, of course, is that it is far safer to purchase your own professional liability insurance policy.

Key Features of a Private Policy

If an employer's liability insurance policy has its limitations, how exactly does a private professional liability policy differ? How expensive is it? And what kind of additional protection does such a policy really provide? Always examine the key features of an insurance policy before signing anything, and know ahead of time what features you should expect to find (Figure 9-2).

Cost

A good place to start is with cost. The good news is that a professional liability policy for an employed healthcare professional is generally fairly inexpensive. For such a low cost and the protection that the policy affords, most professionals feel it is worth the peace of mind to not take the risk of practicing without such a policy.

Disciplinary Defense Insurance

One important feature that comes with many private policies is the additional bonus of disciplinary defense insurance as part of the package. Disciplinary defense

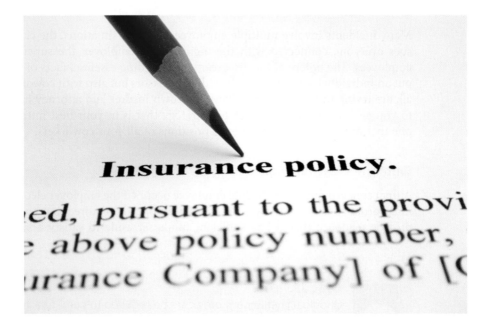

Figure 9-2 Always examine the key features of an insurance policy before signing anything, and know ahead of time what features you should expect to find.

insurance will pay expenses for healthcare providers who must defend themselves in a disciplinary action before a state regulatory board. The policy routinely covers costs of having qualified attorneys represent clients. This additional policy may also cover the following:

1. Legal fee reimbursement/attorney fees
2. Reimbursement for loss of wages
3. Reimbursement for travel, food, and lodging

Policy Limits

Most practitioners select professional liability policies with a limit of $1 million per malpractice incident and a limit of $3 million total ("in aggregate") to be paid over the period the policy is in place. However, insurers do offer higher limits, and practitioners should discuss their particular practices with a representative to determine the coverage level that is appropriate.

Coverage

Commonly, the employer's policy excludes protection for its employees for cases such as quasi-intentional torts of libel or slander and for intentional acts, such as assault and battery. If a claim is made against an employer for acts of this nature by an employee, the employee in that case would receive no help from the employer's insurer for services such as providing legal counsel to the employee in negotiations, mediations, or arbitrations with the claimant; offering representation in court proceedings; filing court documents; investigating the alleged incident; and advising the employee regarding case strategy.

Peace of Mind

The benefit of knowing that you have someone on your side if you are ever involved in a claim against you is priceless. The insurer provides an attorney to assist you in your defense. Also, if a judgment is awarded against you, the insurance company pays the money award to the plaintiff, up to and including the limits of your policy. It will not come out of your pocket.

What If?

You are driving to a patient's home to render services and you are involved in a motor vehicle accident. You are given a ticket because you ran a red light. The driver in the other car is severely injured.

1. Who is likely to be sued?
2. Can your employer be held liable?

Applying for Professional Liability Insurance

To help with the selection of the correct policy provisions and limits of coverage, an insurer will take into account an individual healthcare provider's situation. An applicant must be thorough and honest in providing information to the insurance representative. If you are an independent contractor, inform the representative of the details of your practice and job description including, but not limited to, those described in the following box.

Details to Provide When Applying for Professional Liability Insurance

1. What services do you provide?

   Inform the representative in writing about your typical day-to-day duties and those services that you provide on rare occasions, as well as those that you do not provide now but are considering in the future. This prevents denial of coverage by your insurer because of your concealment or misrepresentation if an incident occurs while performing a service you did not previously mention. Also, the representative will take your specific occupation into account. For example, some services provided by a physical therapist have a higher incidence of related claims than most of those provided by a medical records technician.

2. What types of clients do you serve?

   For example, are the clients frail, elderly, children, or disabled?

3. Do you employ or supervise others, even if only occasionally?

4. Are you supervised and by whom?

   Supervision may affect the independent contractor status.

5. Are you in compliance with all licensing requirements, if required in your state?

6. Have you ever had a lawsuit or disciplinary action filed against you?

7. Are there any incidents that have occurred in the past that could possibly give rise to a future claim?

8. Did the incident occur during the course and scope of employment?

Types of Private Liability Policies

A practitioner's liability insurance policy is tailored to fit a specific type of practice. However, the provisions typically include the elements discussed subsequently.

At the beginning of the policy form, there is usually a statement that identifies your policy as either a claims-made or an occurrence basis policy.

A claims-made policy means that coverage is provided for any claim made while the policy is in effect. For example, you purchase a claims-made policy with coverage from March 1, 2013, through March 1, 2014, but at the end of that term you decide not to renew because you are no longer employed as a healthcare provider. If a claim is made against you on March 1, 2014, coverage applies. However, if the incident triggering the claim occurred during the policy period on March 1, 2013, but the claim was not made against you until June 1, 2014, there is usually no coverage under this policy, unless you have purchased tail coverage (discussed next).

Some policies provide that if you notify your insurer before the expiration of the policy of an incident that you believe could evolve into a claim, then coverage is provided. Also, many policies provide, at no extra charge, a 60-day extension following expiration of the policy during which the insurer will defend you in a claim filed during that 60-day period. If neither of these two modifications for coverage exists, then you should consider purchasing tail coverage.

Tail Coverage

Tail coverage is a special policy that extends the coverage provided in the original policy for a specified period. If in the preceding example you purchased a tail to extend coverage until March 1, 2014, and a claim was made on June 1, 2014, then coverage applies.

Occurrence Basis Policy

An *occurrence basis policy* provides coverage for an incident that occurs during the policy period, regardless of when the claim is made. For example, you purchase an occurrence basis policy with coverage from March 1, 2013, through March 1, 2014, but then decide not to renew the policy. If a claim is made on July 4, 2014, based on an incident that occurred during the policy period, coverage applies. You would not, however, have coverage for any incident that occurred *before* the beginning effective date of the policy unless you purchased prior acts coverage (described below).

Occurrence basis coverage offers the safest protection because you usually know whether an incident will trigger a claim. Insurers are increasingly omitting occurrence policies in favor of claims-made policies. This is probably because the period of time for which an insurer must be concerned about a claim can be definitely determined.

Medical facilities usually obtain occurrence policies. Under such a policy, if you no longer work for the employer, the employer and you still have coverage for an incident that occurred while you were employed. However, if the employer has a claims-made policy, then your coverage depends on the policy provisions. The importance of knowing the provisions in your employer's policy is evident because you should know whether to consider purchasing tail coverage.

Prior Acts Coverage

Another concern with claims-made policies is that they generally do not cover prior acts—those incidents that occurred before the beginning effective date of the policy. Prior acts coverage can be purchased for an additional premium. The insurer issues prior acts coverage going back for a certain period of time. The insurer requires that the professional provide the following information:

1. Services that were provided
2. Whether the professional was employed or self-employed
3. Details regarding any incident that the professional believes might possibly evolve into a claim

Not divulging such information can result in the insurer having no obligation to provide a defense for any claim related to the incident.

Relate to Practice

A patient was treated as an outpatient at a medical facility and prescribed a sulfa drug. The patient was allergic to sulfa drugs, a fact that was noted in the written medical record. However, the medical records technician did not transcribe the allergy note into the computerized patient record. Upon discharge from the facility, the nurse failed to check the written record. The pharmacist who dispensed the drug did not note the allergy. After taking one dose of the sulfa drug, the patient had a severe allergic reaction that ultimately led to her death. The patient's family sued the pharmacist and the facility for the negligence of the nurse and the medical records technician. If the claim against the technician was made after the technician left the facility's employ, did the facility's occurrence-basis liability insurance provide coverage to defend the technician?

Umbrella Policy

The practitioner may also want to consider additional liability protection by purchasing an umbrella policy. The maximum amount payable under a basic liability policy may become exhausted, for example, when there are multiple claims. An umbrella policy provides coverage beyond the amount limits of the basic policy. It may also provide coverage for events excluded from coverage under a basic policy. For example, an umbrella policy may be written to provide coverage for allegations of defamation where there is no such coverage under the basic policy. The amount of coverage desired and the particular events covered determine the cost of an umbrella policy.

Additional Coverage

Finally, insurance companies that provide professional liability insurance may also provide additional coverage, including the following:

1. Defendant expense benefit: reimburses aggregate wages up to a limit and covered expenses incurred when a healthcare provider is on trial as a defendant in a claim covered by insurance.
2. License protection: reimburses up to a limit for defense or disciplinary actions or other covered expenses arising out of an incident covered.
3. Personal liability protection: covers up to limits chosen for liability damages for covered claims unrelated to work resulting from incidents at your personal residence.
4. Medical payments: pays up to the amount determined and reimburses medical expenses to persons injured at your premises or home.
5. Assault coverage: covers medical expenses or property damage and reimburses up to a specific amount per incident if you are assaulted at work or while commuting to and from the workplace.
6. Personal injury protection: protects you up to specified limits against claims of slander, assault, battery, and privacy violation, or other alleged personal injuries committed in the provision of professional services.
7. First aid benefit: reimburses up to a specified amount for expenses incurred from rendering first aid to others.
8. Damage to property of others: pays up to a specified aggregate amount for damage incidents you accidentally cause to others' property.
9. Deposition representation: reimburses up to a specified amount for attorneys' fees for depositions required for incidences arising out of professional services.

Components of a Typical Professional Liability Policy

Suppose you have just acquired a private professional liability policy—or better still, suppose you are about to sign on the dotted line. What should you expect to find? What key components should you look for in the policy document itself?

Declarations Page

The declarations page lists the name(s) of the person or institution insured. It should also list a sum identified as the aggregate limit. This represents the total amount that the insurer will pay during the policy period, usually 1 year, regardless of the number of incidents, claims, claimants, or defendants. For example, if a policy declarations page provides for $3 million of aggregate coverage and $1 million has been used to provide a defense for an incident, then $2 million of coverage remains for the balance of the policy period. This may seem like a large amount, but it can easily be exhausted if several serious incidents occur during the policy period. The declarations page also notes the dates indicating the period of time for which coverage is provided and the premium charged. In the case of an employer's policy, this page also lists the categories of employees who are covered.

This page also describes the limitations of liability. These limitations usually take two forms: (1) per incident or occurrence, and (2) aggregate, with specific dollar amounts noted for each type. *Per incident* (in a health professional's policy it is usually called a *medical incident*) indicates the maximum amount that the insurer will pay to defend a claim that arises from a single incident. For example, suppose the declarations page shows "$1,000,000 per incident." This means that the insurer pays up to that amount only, regardless of the number of claimants or insured involved. *Aggregate limit* refers, as we have seen, to the total amount the policy will pay out over the entire period of coverage.

Policy Provisions

The **policy jacket** is the section that sets forth the generic provisions found in most policies of the same type (Figure 9-3). The provisions are usually separated into

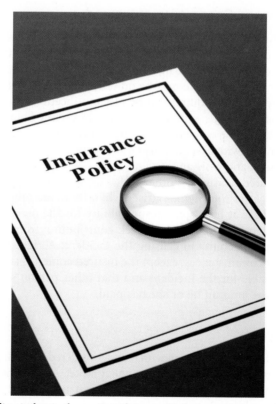

Figure 9-3 The policy jacket is the section that sets forth the generic provisions found in most policies of the same type.

separate sections and generally include the elements discussed in the subsequent sections.

Statement of the Agreement

This statement is often called the **insuring agreement** or **insuring clause** and states the agreement between the insurer and the insured as to what coverage is provided. The clause briefly states what types of claims (e.g., damages due to injury) the insurer is obligated to pay and under what conditions (e.g., injury attributable to acts or omissions of the insured) while the policy is in force.

Exclusions

The **exclusions** section details all the circumstances for which coverage is not provided. Typical examples include, but are not limited to, claims that have the following properties:

1. Allege defamation or discrimination
2. Result from an incident that occurred before the beginning date of the policy
3. Result from an injury the insured either expected or intended
4. Arise under any contract the insured has in which the insured agrees to assume the liability of others
5. Arise out of the commission of a criminal act
6. Arise out of sexual misconduct with a patient or sexual assault

Duties and Cooperation of Insured

The duties and cooperation section lists the duties and required cooperation of the insured in the event of a claim and/or incident. It states how soon after a claim the insured must notify the insurer. Sometimes this is a specific number of days, but commonly the time frame may be quite vague, saying "as soon as practicable." There may or may not be a requirement that the notification be in writing. However, the prudent professional sends written notification by certified mail with a return receipt requested. In addition, the cooperation of the insured also usually includes assistance in securing and giving evidence, attendance at hearings and trials, help securing the attendance of witnesses, and assistance in enforcing any right of "contribution" or "indemnity" that the insured has against others.

A *right of contribution* arises when there are others who, though not named in a claim, bear at least some responsibility for the incident. The insured, if found liable, has a right in some states to seek contribution from others based on a percentage of their responsibility in causing the incident. A right to **indemnification** arises under similar circumstances, except the insured contends that some other person was totally responsible for the incident and that other person should reimburse the insured for the entire amount he or she has paid.

Definitions

All of the words in a policy that are considered insurance terms that the average person may not know are defined in the policy jacket. Also defined are those terms that the insurer wants to be sure that the courts will construe in a certain way if a question of coverage arises. Such words as *medical incidents, claim, injury,* and even *you* are usually defined.

Nonrenewal or Cancellation

The nonrenewal or cancellation section describes the conditions under which the insurer can elect to not renew or to cancel the policy. Usually, the insurer does not need to have a reason. However, there are generally requirements for providing notice to the insured. Typically, if the insurer is not renewing the policy, it must notify the insured in writing at least 30 days before the policy expiration date. If the insurer plans to cancel the policy, most policy provisions state that it must provide written notice at least 10 days before cancellation for nonpayment of the premium and at least 30 days before cancellation if for any other reason.

Right to Defend or Settle

In this section, the insurer states its duty to defend claims as well as its right to do so, even if the facts indicate that the claim has no merit or appears to be fraudulent. This is the section where the insurer may also state that it has a right to settle a claim, if it determines that settlement is appropriate, without the permission of the insured. One reason the insurer may offer settlement to a claimant is that it believes the claimant has a plausible claim that may result in a high jury award if litigated. Also, the claimant may offer to settle for an amount that the insurer believes is less than the claimant might receive if he or she prevails at trial. In either case, the insured may have little or no input in the decision, even if the insured believes that he or she has done nothing wrong.

Other Insurance

Typically, the other insurance section addresses how the payment of claims is affected if there is other insurance available to pay a given claim. This situation arises when, for example, an employer's policy and a second (e.g., professional's individual) policy provide coverage for a single medical incident. The employer's policy may state that it will only apply coverage after the second policy's limits have been paid. The amount the insurer is obligated to pay after the second policy has been paid is called excess coverage. If the second policy has the same provision, so that both policies are excess coverage, then the two insurers will generally share equally in the total amount paid to defend the claim.

Expenses of Defending a Claim

Some policies provide that the expenses (e.g., attorneys' fees, expert witness fees) are included in the limits of liability amounts. This reduces the amount available to pay the claimant's damages, regardless of whether the damages are determined by settlement, mediation, or arbitration. Other policies provide that expenses are paid over and above whatever the claimant actually receives.

Premium Payments

Usually, the premium section does not provide information regarding the time, method, or amount of the premium but states that the rates are in accordance with those in effect at the time and that the premiums are payable when they become due. As discussed earlier, an insurer generally cannot cancel a policy for default in premium payment until it has provided to the insured a timely notice of premium due and intent to cancel before cancellation.

Endorsements

The policy usually contains added provisions that delete or modify the coverage provided in the standard provisions or policy jacket section. These provisions, sometimes called *riders,* address items that apply to the insured's specific situation. For example, there may be a provision that the insurer pays for expenses resulting from the insured being the victim of an assault while at work or possibly while traveling to and from work. The insurer may provide coverage for claims based on defamation or other nonmedical incidents. The insurer may grant an option to the insured to extend liability coverage (i.e., to purchase tail coverage) upon termination of the policy. A rider may also be purchased to cover specific jobs or services the healthcare practitioner provides.

Conclusion: Before Purchasing a Policy

The time to determine what protection a professional liability policy provides is before its purchase, not when a claim is filed. Before purchase, a professional should obtain a sample policy and discuss any questions with the insurance agent. When the policy is issued, the professional should read the entire policy to be sure that it provides the coverage discussed with the agent. Even the most proficient and careful practitioners can be sued when there is no wrongful act or neglect on their part. Having a liability policy ensures that professionals are not subject to the possible economic disaster that can result in defending a claim or having a judgment awarded against them.

Chapter Review Questions

1. _____ is a type of liability insurance that provides coverage beyond the payment amount limits of the basic policy and provides coverage for events excluded from coverage under a basic policy.
   A. Tail coverage
   B. Umbrella coverage
   C. Prior acts coverage
   D. Self-insurance

2. _____ is typically excluded from an employer's liability insurance.
   A. Libel
   B. Negligence
   C. Malpractice
   D. All of the above

3. Which legal theory is similar to the theory of *respondeat superior*?
   A. Quasi-intentional tort
   B. Occurrence basis policy
   C. Vicarious liability
   D. Negligence

4. Which type of liability policy provides coverage for an incident that occurs during the policy period, regardless of when the claim is made?
   A. Claim-based policy
   B. Prior acts coverage
   C. Tail coverage
   D. Occurrence basis policy

5. Which section of a liability insurance policy lists the amount of coverage?
   A. Declarations page
   B. Statement of the agreement
   C. Exclusions section
   D. Definitions section

Self-Reflection Questions

1. Why do you, as a healthcare professional, need professional liability insurance?
2. Why is it important to know the coverage of your employer's liability insurance as well as coverage it excludes?

Internet Activities

1. Search the Internet and find two companies writing policies for your area of practice.
2. Search the Internet or discuss disciplinary actions that have been taken against healthcare providers in your field.
3. Search the Internet and discuss a case based on medical malpractice in your field

Bibliography

Dobbyn JF: *Insurance law*, St Paul, Minn, 1989, West Publishing, pp 152-160.
Glannon JW: *The law of torts*, Boston, 1995, Little, Brown, pp 375-378.
Harris County Hosp. Dist. v. Estrada, 872 S.W.2d 729 (Tex. 1993).
Prosser W: *Handbook of the law of torts*, St Paul, Minn, 1975, West Publishing, pp 468-475.
Id. at 458-459.
Prosser, *supra* note 1, at 305-313.
Smith JW: *Hospital liability,* § 5.01(7), New York, 1998, Law Journal Seminars-Press.
Smith, *supra* note 3, at § 5.02(3).
Smith, *supra* note 3, at § 5.01(3).
Smith, *supra* note 3, at § 5.01(6).
Id. at § 5.01(7).
www.naplia.com.
www.imri.com.

Chapter 10

Death and Dying Issues

Christopher Lee

KEY TERMS

Active euthanasia The active acceleration of death by the use of drugs, for example, whether by oneself or with the aid of a physician.

Advance directive The treatment preferences and designation of an alternate decision maker in the event that a person should become unable to make medical decisions on his or her own behalf.

Brain death The irreversible loss of function of the brain, including the brain stem.

Death The permanent cessation of all biological functions that sustain a living organism.

Durable power of attorney A type of advance medical directive in which legal documents provide the power of attorney to another person in the case of an incapacitating medical condition.

Euthanasia Termination of a life to eliminate pain and suffering related to a terminal illness, usually performed by giving a drug or agent to induce cessation of body functions. Also known as assisted suicide.

Healthcare proxy A legal document in which an individual designates another person to make healthcare decisions if he or she is rendered incapable of making his or her wishes known.

Hospice Organization or program involving a multidisciplinary group of medical professionals available to aid in support of the terminally ill and their families.

Involuntary euthanasia The active effort to end the life of a patient who has not explicitly requested aid in dying. This term is most often used with respect to patients who are in a persistent vegetative state and who probably will never recover consciousness.

Living will A document in which the patient states his or her wishes regarding medical treatment, especially treatment that sustains or prolongs life by extraordinary means, in the event that the patient becomes mentally incompetent or unable to communicate.

National Organ Transplant Act (NOTA) Act of Congress that established the Organ Procurement and Transplantation Network (OPTN) to maintain a national registry for organ matching and to provide grants to qualified organ procurement organizations.

Passive euthanasia The act of allowing a patient to die without medical intervention.

Patient Self-Determination Act Federal law that requires all healthcare institutions receiving Medicare or Medicaid funds to provide patients with written information about their right under state law to execute advance directives. The written information must clearly state the institution's policies on withholding or withdrawing life-sustaining treatment.

Persistent vegetative state (PVS) Condition characterized by the irreversible cessation of higher brain functions, usually as a result of damage to the cerebral cortex.

Terminally ill Illness with an expected survival of less than 6 months.

Thanatology The study of the effects of death and dying, especially the investigation of ways to lessen the suffering and address the needs of the terminally ill and their survivors.

Uniform Anatomical Gift Act Legislation that allows a person to make an anatomical gift at the time of death by the use of a signed document such as a will or driver's license—the person can donate all or part of his or her body for medical education, scientific research, or organ transplantation.

Uniform Determination of Death Act (UDDA) Model state legislation that has since been adopted by most U.S. states and is intended "to provide a comprehensive and medically sound basis for determining death in all situations."

Uniform Rights of the Terminally Ill Act Legislation that allows a person to declare a living will specifying that, if the situation arises, he or she does not wish to be kept alive through life support if terminally ill or in a coma. The patient may also obtain a healthcare power of attorney. This power of attorney appoints an agent to make medical decisions for the patient in case the patient becomes incompetent.

Voluntary euthanasia Conscious medical act that results in the death of a patient who has given consent.

CHAPTER OBJECTIVES

1. Define death and describe the criteria for determination of death set forth in the UDDA.
2. List the threshold criteria for determining brain death.
3. Identify stages of grief.
4. Define and differentiate various advance medical directives, including the difference between an advance directive, a living will, a durable power of attorney, a healthcare proxy, and a DNR order.
5. Identify the functions of hospice.
6. Delineate the various kinds of euthanasia and the controversy surrounding this issue, including landmark court decisions.
7. Discuss the process for organ donation.

Introduction

Death is the permanent ending of all biological functions that sustain a living organism. Common causes that bring about death include aging, malnutrition, disease, suicide, murder, and accidents or trauma resulting in terminal injury. In most human societies, the nature of death has for centuries been a topic of religious traditions and of philosophical and scientific study. These approaches may include a belief in some kind of resurrection or reincarnation or the idea that consciousness simply ceases to exist. In fact, scientific interest has led to development of the field of thanatology, which is devoted to the study of effects of death and dying.

Death affects not only the one who dies but also those who remain behind, typically producing feelings of grief or emotional suffering associated with having something or someone that is loved, valued, and/or cherished taken away. After death, there may be various mourning or funeral practices, in accordance with the individual's personal religious or social beliefs.

Even from a purely scientific viewpoint, we encounter numerous approaches to the concept of death, and attempts to define the exact moment of a human's death have proved problematic. Death was once defined as the absence of a heartbeat and breathing, but the development of cardiopulmonary resuscitation (CPR) and prompt defibrillation have rendered that definition useless because breathing and heartbeat can sometimes be restarted. In addition, events that were once likely causes of death no longer kill in all situations. Even without a functioning heart or lungs, life can sometimes be sustained with a combination of life-support devices, organ transplants, and artificial pacemakers. Finally, our understanding of the brain raises questions of what makes us human and alive. For example, patients who sustain damage to their cerebral cortex may fall into a persistent vegetative state (PVS), in which the individual may have moments of assumed wakefulness and reflexive responses, but has permanently lost the higher functions of the brain. Only autonomic or involuntary processes remain. Needless to say, viewing a loved one in such a state can raise conflicting feelings among family members regarding whether or not the person is truly "there" and "alive."

Determination of Death

So, in such increasingly complex medical states and treatments, how does a physician determine the moment of death? Today, when a definition of the moment of death is required, physicians usually turn to "brain death" or "biological death" to define a person as being dead; people are considered dead when the electrical activity in their brain ceases. In an effort to provide medical professionals with a more consistent definition of death and to provide guidelines for the determination of death, the Uniform Determination of Death Act (UDDA) was approved in 1981. The UDDA is a draft state law that was approved for the United States by the National Conference of Commissioners on Uniform State Laws, in cooperation with the American Medical Association, the American Bar Association, and the President's Commission for the Study of Ethical Problems in Medicine and Biomedical and Behavioral Research. It has since been adopted by most U.S. states and is intended "to provide a comprehensive and medically sound basis for determining death in all situations." For legal purposes, the UDDA states that for determination of death, an individual who has sustained either (1) irreversible interruption of circulatory and respiratory functions, or (2) irreversible interruption of all functions of the entire brain, including the brain stem, is dead.

However, that second part still raises challenges. The determination of brain death can be complicated, and a determination of death must be made in accordance with accepted medical standards. It is presumed that an end of electrical activity indicates the end of consciousness. However, absence of consciousness must be permanent, and not transient as occurs during certain sleep stages, and especially a coma. In the case of sleep, electroencephalograms (EEGs) can easily tell the difference by detecting spurious electrical impulses, while certain drugs, hypoglycemia, hypoxia, or hypothermia can suppress or even stop brain activity temporarily. Because of this, hospitals have protocols for determining brain death involving EEGs at widely separated intervals under defined conditions. There are also certain criteria that need to be met before a patient can be pronounced brain dead, including the following:

- No pupil response
- No blinking reflex
- No grimace reflex
- No response to pain
- No coughing or gagging reflex
- No unassisted breathing

If these criteria have been met, then the patient fulfills one or both of the qualifications established in the UDDA and is therefore considered dead.

Grief

Grief is a natural response to any significant loss. It is the emotional suffering one feels when something or someone the individual loves is taken away. The grief associated with death is familiar to most people, but individuals grieve in connection with a variety of losses throughout their lives, such as unemployment, ill health, or the end of a relationship. Loss can be categorized as either physical or abstract, the physical loss being related to something that the individual can touch or measure, such as losing a spouse through death, whereas other types of loss are abstract, and relate to aspects of a person's social interactions.

In 1969, psychologist Elisabeth Kübler-Ross introduced her hypothesis regarding grief and grieving in her book *On Death and Dying*. In it, she describes the "five stages of grief." Her hypothesis proposed that both the individual facing the reality of impending death and also those who care about them tend to experience a series of fairly predictable emotional "stages" of grief: denial, anger, bargaining, depression, and acceptance (in no specific sequence) (Figure 10-1). The stages, popularly known by the acronym DABDA, include:

- **Denial**—Denial is usually only a temporary defense for the patient. The patient may initially be unable to accept that his or her condition is terminal and that death is inevitable. This feeling is generally replaced with heightened awareness of possessions and individuals who will be left behind after death.
- **Anger**—In the second stage, the patient recognizes that denial cannot continue. Anger can manifest itself in different ways. People can be angry with themselves, or with others, and especially those who are close to them.
- **Bargaining**—In the third stage, the patient hopes to somehow postpone or delay death. Usually, the negotiation for an extended life is made with a higher power in exchange for a reformed lifestyle.
- **Depression**—During the fourth stage, the patient begins to understand that death is certain and imminent. Because of this, the patient may become silent, refuse visitors, and spend much of the time crying and grieving. This is actually an essential and helpful process that allows the dying person to disconnect from things of love and affection and makes way for a sense of acceptance. It is natural to feel sadness, regret, fear, and uncertainty when going through this stage. Feeling those emotions shows that the person has begun to accept the situation.
- **Acceptance**—In this last stage, the patient may begin to come to terms with his or her mortality, or that of a loved one, or other tragic event. This stage varies according to the person's situation. People dying can enter this stage a long time before the people they leave behind, who must pass through their own individual stages of dealing with the grief.

Kübler-Ross noted that these stages are not meant to be a complete list of all possible emotions that could be felt, and can occur in any order. Her hypothesis also states that not everyone who experiences a loss feels all five of the responses, since reactions to personal losses of any kind are as unique as the person experiencing them.

Advance Medical Directives

Advancements in technology and medicine have enabled healthcare providers to resuscitate patients in cardiac or respiratory arrest as well as maintain their life indefinitely with support measures. However, not all patients wish for these measures to be taken.

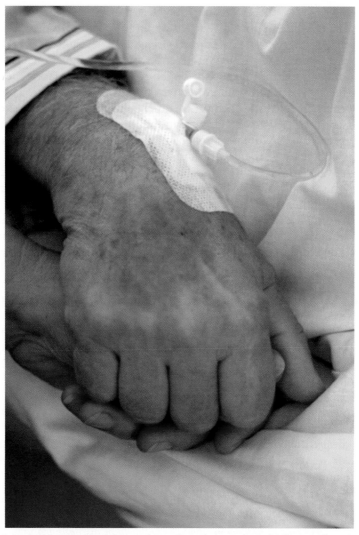

Figure 10-1 Both the individual facing the reality of impending death as well as those who care about the individual tend to experience a series of fairly predictable emotional "stages" of grief.

The **Uniform Rights of the Terminally Ill Act** states that all patients have the right to create a living will to make their wishes known in the event they are incapacitated as well as designate alternate decision makers through a healthcare proxy or durable power of attorney. In 1990, the federal government passed the **Patient Self-Determination Act (PSDA)**. This legislation mandates that hospitals, nursing homes, hospice providers, and other healthcare agencies provide written information to patients regarding their rights to make medical decisions and execute advance directives. The requirements of the PSDA are as follows:

Patients are given written notice upon admission to the healthcare facility of their decision-making rights, and policies regarding advance healthcare directives in their state and in the institution to which they have been admitted. Patient rights include the following:

- The right to facilitate their own healthcare decisions
- The right to accept or refuse medical treatment
- The right to make an advance healthcare directive

Advance directives are usually written documents designed to allow competent patients the opportunity to guide future healthcare decisions in the event that they are unable to participate directly in medical decision making. The term "advance directives" refers to treatment preferences and the designation of a surrogate decision maker in the event that a person should become unable to make medical decisions on her or his own behalf. Advance directives are designed to outline a person's wishes and preferences in regard to medical treatments and interventions, and to identify a potential healthcare proxy—that is, an individual the person authorizes to act on the patient's behalf (in case the person becomes incapacitated or unable to communicate) to make decisions consistent with and based on the patient's stated will. Drafting a proper advance directive form may require assistance from a physician and/or an attorney. This is especially noteworthy since advance directive policies may differ from one state to another.

Facilities must inquire as to whether the patient has an advance healthcare directive, and make note of this in the patient's medical records. They must also provide education to their staff and affiliates about these directives. Healthcare providers are not allowed to discriminately admit or treat patients based on whether or not they have an advance healthcare directive. Finally, it is important to note that an individual's wishes expressed in an advance directive supersede those of the family or significant other. Below are a few more key points to keep in mind when arranging for—or helping a patient arrange for—an advance directive:

Advance directives generally fall into three categories: living will, healthcare proxy, and durable power of attorney.

Living Will

This is a written document that specifies what types of medical treatment are desired should the individual become incapacitated. A living will can be general or very specific. The most common statement in a living will is usually something similar to this:

> *"If I suffer an incurable, irreversible illness, disease, or condition and my attending physician determines that my condition is terminal, I direct that life-sustaining measures that would serve only to prolong my dying be withheld or discontinued."*

More specific living wills may include information regarding an individual's desire for services such as the following:

- Analgesia (pain relief)
- Antibiotics
- Artificial (intravenous or IV) hydration
- Artificial feeding (feeding tube)
- CPR (cardiopulmonary resuscitation)
- Life-support equipment including ventilators (breathing machines)
- Do not resuscitate (DNR) order

Healthcare Proxy

This is a legal document in which an individual designates another person to make healthcare decisions if he or she is rendered incapable of making his or her wishes known. The healthcare proxy has, in essence, the same rights to request or refuse treatment that the individual would have if capable of making and communicating decisions.

Durable Power of Attorney (DPOA)

Through this type of advance directive, an individual executes legal documents that provide the power of attorney to others in the case of an incapacitating medical condition. The durable power of attorney allows an individual to make bank transactions, sign Social Security checks, apply for disability, or simply write checks to pay the utility bill while an individual is medically incapacitated.

DPOA can also specifically designate different individuals to act on a person's behalf for specific affairs. For example, one person can be designated the DPOA of healthcare or medical power of attorney, similar to the healthcare proxy, whereas another individual can be made the legal DPOA.

Do Not Resuscitate (DNR)

A *"do not resuscitate"* or *"DNR,"* sometimes called a "No Code," is a legal order written either in the hospital or on a legal form to respect the wishes of a patient to not undergo CPR or advanced cardiac life support (ACLS) if the patient's heart stopped or the patient stopped breathing.

This introduces an important distinction. How does a DNR differ from an advance directive or a living will? It is a matter of authorization. Advance directives and living wills are documents written by individuals themselves, in order to state their wishes for care if they are no longer able to speak for themselves. In contrast, it is a physician or hospital staff member who writes a DNR "physician's order," which is based upon the wishes previously expressed by the patient in his or her advance directive or living will. Likewise, at a time when the patient is unable to express his or her wishes, but has previously used a healthcare proxy advance directive to appoint an alternate decision maker, then a physician can write such a DNR order at the request of the alternate decision maker.

A DNR does not affect any treatment other than that which would require intubation or CPR. Patients who have a DNR order can continue to get chemotherapy, antibiotics, dialysis, or any other appropriate treatments.

What if?
You witness a comatose patient's family member tell the attending physician that the family wishes the patient to be a "DNR." You do not know if the patient has a living will on file or if the patient has a healthcare proxy naming this family member their decision maker. What do you do?

Relate to Practice
Andrew is a medical assistant working in a busy emergency department (ED). An ambulance crew arrives with an elderly man who has been to the ED several times before and has a DNR on file at the hospital. The patient goes into respiratory arrest, but his daughter states that the family wants all life-saving measures taken, regardless of the DNR on file. What should Andrew do?

Relate to Practice

One role of medical assistants in healthcare is to provide patient education. Jeanette has been a medical assistant in internal medicine for 7 years with Dr. Willet. The medical office serves mainly older high-risk patients; therefore, it is customary practice to discuss and educate patients on the importance of advance directives, living will, and power of attorney. At the request of Dr. Willet, Jeanette is asked to temporarily assist at Glendale Summit Medical Clinic. Jeanette is aware the clientele is different from her current office. Here, many of the patients are much younger, and a significant number are from lower socioeconomic backgrounds. She relishes this change and is enthusiastic about expanding her experience with this new population. At the request of the office manager, Jeanette assists in auditing patient charts. She notices many patients do not have advance directives on file. For Jeanette, this is a serious cause for concern.

1. Why do you think this is a serious concern for Jeanette? Should this truly be her concern?
2. How should Jeanette approach this concern? And with whom?
3. The head physician decides to incorporate advance directive patient education for new and existing patients. Jeanette is asked to supply information for distribution. What resources are available for her to use? Where can they be found?

Hospice

In many chronic and progressive conditions such as cancer, heart disease, or dementia, as a disease progresses to an advanced stage, its symptoms become more intolerable and difficult to control. As a result, an end-stage condition can significantly impair a person's functional status and quality of life. In addition, at such a point, aggressive treatments may offer little benefit while posing significant risk and jeopardizing the patient's well-being. At this point, often there is no further cure or treatment to control the progression of the disease.

In such late stages of diseases, especially when there is "nothing left to do," hospice can offer help for patients and families (Figure 10-2). Hospice care promotes open discussions about "the big picture" with patients and their loved ones. The disease process, prognosis, and realities are often important parts of these discussions. More importantly, the patient's wishes, values, and beliefs are taken into account and become the cornerstone of the hospice plan of care.

Most people are familiar with the term hospice as a place to receive care for the terminally ill patient. In some cases, hospice can involve a specific facility or location, but strictly speaking, hospice is a service, rather than a physical place, that provides palliative care for patients in the late stages of a terminal illness. A hospice team consists of physicians, nurses, social workers, clerics, volunteers, and therapists, who work together with the common goal to provide comfort, reduce suffering, and preserve patient dignity, as well as provide emotional support for the family and caregiver. Medicare, Medicaid, and most private insurance carriers provide hospice benefits. Some people have the mistaken notion that hospice is used to hasten or prolong death, but as more people now are seeing hospice as a frequent choice for more and more individuals, the hope is that this misconception will soon disappear.

Patients and families who transfer into hospice find themselves served by a team who focuses on providing a peaceful, symptom-free, and dignified transition to death

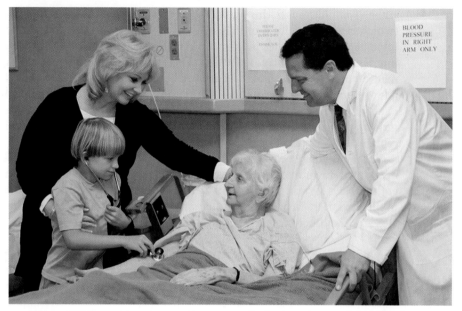

Figure 10-2 Hospice care provides support for both patients and their loved ones.

for patients whose diseases are advanced beyond a cure. The hope for a cure shifts to hope for a life free of suffering. The focus becomes quality of life rather than its length.

The complex care of hospice patients may include the following:

- Managing evolving medical issues (e.g., infections, medication management, pressure ulcers, hydration, nutrition, physical stages of dying)
- Treating physical symptoms (e.g., pain, shortness of breath, anxiety, nausea, vomiting, constipation, confusion)
- Counseling about the anxiety, uncertainty, grief, and fear associated with end of life and dying
- Rendering support to patients, their families, and caregivers with the overwhelming physical and psychological stresses of a terminal illness
- Guiding patients and families through the difficult interpersonal and psychosocial issues and helping them with finding closure
- Paying attention to personal, religious, spiritual, and cultural values
- Assisting patients and families reaching financial closures (living will, trust, advance directive, funeral arrangements)
- Providing bereavement counseling to the mourning loved ones after the death of the patient

 Discussion
Why is it important for hospice to integrate the patient's family into the hospice experience?

Euthanasia

Euthanasia, from the Greek term meaning "good death," refers to the practice of intentionally ending a life in order to relieve pain and suffering through medical means. It is important to note that the word "intentionally" is key to the definition of euthanasia. Although this definition is strikingly similar to premeditated murder (which is why it is illegal in many U.S. states and countries throughout the world), the important difference lies in the reasoning behind the intent: to relieve pain and suffering. This seeming contradiction has created debate among bioethicists, psychologists, medical professionals, and the general population for decades. The topic of euthanasia is extremely controversial, and there are numerous arguments on both sides of the issue. Over the years, there have been a number of movements, organizations, societies, articles, campaigns, books, speeches, and even films dedicated to this issue, and yet it remains unresolved.

Euthanasia may be classified according to whether a person gives informed consent, breaking it down into three types: voluntary, nonvoluntary, and involuntary. Voluntary euthanasia is legal in some countries and U.S. states. Nonvoluntary euthanasia is illegal in all countries. Involuntary euthanasia is usually considered murder. We will look closer at the differences.

- Voluntary euthanasia: euthanasia conducted with the consent and participation of the patient
- Nonvoluntary euthanasia: euthanasia conducted when the consent of the patient is unavailable or unattained.
- Involuntary euthanasia: euthanasia conducted against the wishes of the patient or the patient's surrogate decision maker

Passive and Active Euthanasia

Voluntary, nonvoluntary, and involuntary euthanasia can all be further divided into passive or active. Passive euthanasia entails the withholding of common treatments, such as antibiotics, necessary for survival. This ensures that the patient dies "naturally." Active euthanasia is much more controversial and entails the conscious use of lethal substances or forces, such as administering a lethal injection.

Physician-Assisted Suicide

Euthanasia that is conducted or carried out in the presence of or with the cooperation of a physician is termed physician-assisted suicide. This is legal in some countries, whereas in the United States the debate over a patient's right to die was brought to the forefront through the controversial work of Dr. Kevorkian, a physician who developed two types of devices that enabled patients to participate in voluntary euthanasia for end-of-life conditions. With each device, administering the final dose was left up to the patient to provide maximum control of his or her own death. Dr. Kevorkian was eventually convicted and served 8 years for second-degree murder. He was released on condition that he would not advise anyone else on how to commit suicide. Kevorkian once said of his work: "My aim in helping the patient was not to cause death. My aim was to end suffering. It's got to be decriminalized."

Landmark Court Decisions Related to Death and Dying

There have been three landmark court decisions that have had significant impact on the issues of euthanasia, right to die, and advance directives. These court decisions continue to affect the lives of terminally ill patients today. All of these decisions were controversial and are, in fact, still the subject of debate. However, they have laid much of the legal framework we use in making many end-of-life decisions.

Karen Ann Quinlan

The case of Karen Ann Quinlan was an important precedent in the history of the right-to-die controversy in the United States. When she was 21, Quinlan became unconscious after arriving home from a party. After she collapsed and stopped breathing twice for 15 minutes or more, the paramedics arrived and took her to a hospital, where she lapsed into a persistent vegetative state. She was kept alive on a ventilator for several months, but showed no improvement. Her parents requested that the hospital discontinue active care and allow her to die. The hospital refused, and the subsequent legal battles made newspaper headlines and set significant precedents. The New Jersey Supreme Court eventually ruled in her parents' favor. Although Quinlan was removed from a ventilator in 1976, she continued to survive in a persistent vegetative state for almost a decade until her death from pneumonia in 1985.

Quinlan's case continues to raise important questions in bioethics, euthanasia, and legal guardianship. Her case has affected the practice of medicine and law around the world. There are two significant outcomes that arose from her case: (1) the development of formal ethics committees in hospitals, nursing homes, and hospices, and (2) the development of advance health directives are both a direct result of *In re Quinlan*.

Nancy Cruzan

In 1983, Nancy Cruzan lost control of her car, was thrown from it, and landed face down in a water-filled ditch. Paramedics found her with no vital signs, but they resuscitated her. After a couple weeks of remaining dormant within a coma, Nancy was diagnosed as being in a persistent vegetative state. A feeding tube was inserted for her long-term care. Her husband and parents waited for a more substantial recovery, but after 4 years, they accepted that there was no hope. The accident occurred 7 years before the parents and husband presented their case to the United States Supreme Court. The issue of this case was whether the State of Missouri had the right to require "clear and convincing evidence" in order for Cruzan's parents to remove their daughter from life support. In a 5 to 4 decision, the U.S. Supreme Court found in favor of the Missouri Department of Health. However, it upheld the legal standard that competent persons are able to exercise the right to refuse medical treatment under the due process clause. Because there was no "clear and convincing evidence" of what Nancy Cruzan wanted, the Court upheld the state's policy. After the case was decided, the family found proof that Nancy Cruzan would have wanted her life support terminated and eventually won a court order to have her removed from life support. Cruzan died 11 days later on December 26, 1990.

Terri Schiavo

The latest, and possibly most famous, case is that of Terri Schiavo. This case was a legal struggle involving prolonged life support that lasted from 1998 to 2005. At issue was whether to carry out the decision of the husband of Teresa Marie "Terri" Schiavo to terminate life support. After the patient was diagnosed by physicians as being in a persistent vegetative state, a series of highly publicized legal challenges presented by her parents and by state and federal legislative intervention caused a 7-year delay before life support was finally terminated.

Terri Schiavo collapsed in her home in full cardiac arrest in 1990. She suffered massive brain damage from lack of oxygen, and after $2\frac{1}{2}$ months in a coma, her diagnosis was changed to persistent vegetative state. Over the next few years, speech and physical therapy and other experimental therapies were attempted, hoping to return her to a state of awareness. In 1998 Michael Schiavo petitioned the Sixth Circuit Court of Florida to remove her feeding tube pursuant to Florida law. He was opposed by Terri's parents, Robert and Mary Schindler, who argued that she was conscious. The court determined that Terri would not wish to continue life-prolonging measures, and on April 24, 2001, her feeding tube was removed for the first time, only to be reinserted several days later. On February 25, 2005, a judge ordered the removal of Terri Schiavo's feeding tube. Several appeals and incidents of federal government intervention followed, which included U.S. President George W. Bush returning to Washington, DC, to sign legislation designed to keep Terri alive. After all attempts at appeals through the federal court system upheld the original decision to remove the feeding tube, staff at the hospice facility where Terri was receiving care disconnected the feeding tube on March 18, 2005, and Terri died on March 31, 2005.

In all, the Schiavo case involved 14 appeals and numerous motions, petitions, and hearings in the Florida courts; 5 suits in federal district court; Florida legislation struck down by the Supreme Court of Florida; federal legislation; and 4 refusals to take up the case from the United States Supreme Court. The case also spurred highly visible activism from the pro-life movement and disability rights groups.

Organ and Tissue Donation

Every year, thousands of people die while waiting for an organ donation that could save their lives. To address the nation's critical organ donation shortage and improve the organ matching and placement process, the U.S. Congress passed the National Organ Transplant Act (NOTA) in 1984. The act established the Organ Procurement and Transplantation Network (OPTN) to maintain a national registry for organ matching (Figure 10-3). Last year alone, organ donations made more than 28,000 transplants possible. Another 1 million people received cornea and other tissue transplants that helped them recover from trauma, bone damage, spinal injuries, burns, hearing impairment, and vision loss. Before the NOTA was enacted, there was no clear jurisdiction on the property rights for a human corpse. Instead, America applied a "quasi-right" to a corpse. This meant that the relatives of a deceased person had a possessory right long enough to decide how to bury or dispose of the corpse. This is not a property right, which means that relatives do not have a right to transfer, devise, possess, and lease the human organs and tissues.

Because of a shortage in organs but a growing demand for transplantations, people began to use other means to purchase organs outside of a hospital setting. The organ market began to become a commercial market. In 1983, H. Barry Jacobs, the head of a Virginia company, announced a new plan to buy and sell human organs on the market. This plan put healthy, human kidneys in the price range of up to $10,000 plus a $20,000 to $50,000 commission fee for Jacobs. This brought the issue out into the open. Passage of NOTA then made it criminal to market for profit human organs for the purposes of a human transplantation.

The Uniform Anatomical Gift Act allows a person to make an anatomical gift at the time of death by the use of a signed document such as a will or driver's license—the person can donate all or part of his or her body for medical education, scientific research, or organ transplantation.

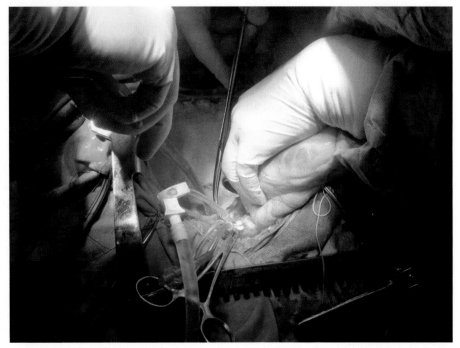

Figure 10-3 The Organ Procurement and Transplantation Network (OPTN) maintains a national registry for organ matching.

Discussion
Do you think that it should be mandatory for everyone to state their wishes regarding organ donation on their driver's license?

Conclusion

Issues surrounding death and dying are numerous and complex. Although some of the more controversial aspects of responding medically to the dying are likely to never be resolved completely, the increasing dialogue on such issues is helping us all to think more consciously about and become more sensitive to the rights and needs of both dying patients and those who will care for and grieve for them.

Chapter Review Questions

1. Which advance directive allows a person to designate another person to make healthcare decisions if he or she is rendered incapable of making his or her wishes known?
   A. Living will
   B. Durable power of attorney
   C. Healthcare proxy
   D. DNR

2. The law mandating that hospitals, nursing homes, hospice providers, and other healthcare agencies provide written information to patients regarding their rights to make medical decisions and execute advance directives is called the
   A. Uniform Determination of Death Act.
   B. Uniform Anatomical Gift Act.
   C. Patient Self-Determination Act.
   D. Uniform Rights of the Terminally Ill Act.

3. The _____ states that all patients have the right to create a living will to make their wishes known in the event they are incapacitated, as well as to designate alternate decision makers through a healthcare proxy or durable power of attorney.
   A. Uniform Determination of Death Act
   B. Uniform Anatomical Gift Act
   C. Patient Self-Determination Act
   D. Uniform Rights of the Terminally Ill Act

4. An individual who has executed a DNR order typically would not receive
   A. chemotherapy.
   B. antibiotics.
   C. IV fluids.
   D. CPR.

5. A _____ is a form of advance directive that specifies what types of medical treatment are desired should the individual become incapacitated.
   A. living will
   B. healthcare proxy
   C. durable power of attorney
   D. DNR

Self-Reflection Questions

1. Think about a time that you experienced a loss. Looking back, did you go through all five stages of grief? Describe how you handled each stage.
2. Do you or any of your family members have advance directives? If so, do you know what they are or what their wishes would be? If not, do you think that everyone should have advance directives? Why or why not?

Internet Activities

1. Visit www.hospicenet.org. List three questions you should ask when deciding which hospice program is right for your needs.
2. Go to www.helpguide.org/mental/grief_loss.htm. What are three tips to help someone cope with grief?

Additional Resources

www.medterms.com.

www.aan.com/professionals/practice/guidelines/pda/Brain_death_adults.pdf.

www.medicareresources.org/glossary/curative-care/.

http://legal-dictionary.thefreedictionary.com/.

http://optn.transplant.hrsa.gov/policiesAndBylaws/nota.asp.

http://depts.washington.edu/bioethx/topics/advdir.html.

'Jacob Jack' Kevorkian dies; death with dignity proponent remembered, medicalnewstoday.com, 2011 (last update). Retrieved November 10, 2011.

Kübler-Ross E: *On death and dying,* New York, 1968, Routledge, ISBN 0-415-04015-9.

Kübler-Ross E: *On grief and grieving: finding the meaning of grief through the five stages of loss,* New York, 2005, Simon & Schuster Ltd, ISBN 0-7432-6344-8.

Scire P: *Applying grief stages to organizational change. An attributional analysis of Kübler-Ross' model of dying,* Mark R. Brent, Boston, Mass, 2007, Harvard University.

What is the Patient Self-Determination Act? See Legal-HelpMate.

Advance care planning in health care reform legislation: National Hospice and Palliative Care Organization, Alexandria, Va.

In re Quinlan, 70 N.J. 10, 355 A.2d 647 (N.J. 1976).

Cruzan v. Director, Missouri Dept. of Health, 497 U.S. 261 (Mo. 1990).

www.organdonor.gov/legislation/index.html.

Chapter 11

Conflict Management

Christopher Lee

Accommodating Conflict behavior style in which an individual allows the needs of a group or team to supersede the individual's own needs. Also known as "smoothing."

Alternative dispute resolution (ADR) The procedure for settling disputes by means other than litigation.

Arbitration A process using a mediator to resolve a dispute between two parties without using a judge and/or a trial process.

Avoiding Conflict behavior style in which the issue is not addressed at all or is ignored.

"Captain of the ship" doctrine An adaptation from the "borrowed servant rules," as applied to an operating room, which arose in *McConnell v. Williams,* holding the person in charge (e.g., a surgeon) responsible for all under his or her supervision, regardless of whether the "captain" is directly responsible for an alleged error or act of alleged negligence, and despite the assistants' positions as hospital employees.

Collaborating Conflict behavior style in which the needs and goals of the individuals are combined to meet a common goal.

Competing Conflict behavior style in which an individual's own needs are advocated over the needs of others.

Compromising Conflict behavior style in which people give and receive in a series of tradeoffs.

Conflict The mental struggle resulting from incompatible or opposing needs, drives, wishes, or external or internal demands.

Conflict management The long-term management of disputes and conflicts, which may or may not lead to resolution.

Conflict resolution The process of ending a disagreement between two or more people in a constructive fashion for all parties involved.

Disagreement A failure to agree.

Disruptive behavior Personal conduct, whether verbal or physical, that affects or that potentially may affect patient care negatively.

Facilitation The process by which a third party (facilitator) assists in the resolution of a dispute.

Mediation The process by which a neutral third party who is trained in mediation techniques facilitates and assists in resolving a dispute.

Negative conflict Conflict that has devolved into disruptive behaviors or violence.

Negotiation Any communication used in an attempt to achieve a goal, approval, or action by another.

Positive conflict The idea that healthy discussion can happen in the face of a disagreement, regardless of differing personalities, education levels, or responsibilities.

The Joint Commission The organization that accredits hospitals and other healthcare organizations.

1. Define conflict, differentiating between positive and negative conflict.
2. Identify various conflict behavioral styles.
3. Identify the emotional, cognitive, and physical responses to conflict.
4. Define disruptive behavior.
5. Compare and contrast conflict management and conflict resolution.
6. Define alternative dispute resolution.
7. Identify the components of alternative dispute resolution.

Introduction

The healthcare industry is subject to increasing strains resulting from demands for broader access to care, greater accountability, and improved quality of care, while facing more work for less pay, staffing shortages, stiffer regulatory enforcement, and decreased reimbursement. The healthcare professional's typical day involves a race to coordinate resources, provide care, perform procedures, gather data, respond to emergencies, solve problems, and interact with diverse groups of people. As a group, healthcare professionals face more conflict and greater complexity than any other field, regardless of the specific role: physician, midlevel provider, nurse, paramedic, medical assistant, surgical technologist, or pharmacy technician. Healthcare providers must face the challenges of balancing competing interests, philosophies, and training backgrounds; survive the endless quest for adequate resources; and deal with the emotional quality of the work that they do. And yet very few have had the opportunity to learn the skills and processes necessary for negotiating their environments. There is little formal training available in this area, and role models for collaboration and good negotiation are few and far between. As a result, the clinical environment is frequently one of competition, quick fixes, hot tempers, and avoidance tactics. It is little wonder that these strains lead to stress and eventual conflict. Although some level of friction is inevitable in any group setting, it is especially likely in the healthcare arena, where differences of authority and knowledge are common. If treated as a normal consequence of human behavior, minor conflicts can reveal problems and serve as a catalyst for necessary change. However, chronic conflict and unacceptable behavior at any level can breed fear and distrust, making teamwork impossible. Failure to resolve these issues can lead professionals to focus on avoiding trouble, rather than doing everything in their power to protect patients.

What Is Conflict?

Conflict is the internal struggle resulting from incompatible or opposing needs, drives, wishes, or external or internal demands. As opposed to a disagreement, which is simply a failure to agree, a conflict involves a perceived threat to an individual's needs, interests, or concerns as a result of a disagreement. Therefore, conflict is a natural and normal part of human interaction. Conflict has two forms. There is a positive aspect that, when managed effectively, leads to change and progress. Indeed, without conflict, areas for change and improvement would not be identified and thus progress would never be made. However, conflict's negative aspect can lead to violence and counterproductive behavior.

Contributing Factors

Patients and providers alike understand that healthcare delivery is a complex environment. We look closely at some of the key characteristics of healthcare that help to create misunderstandings and disputes:

- Within healthcare, misunderstandings and conflict usually involve several distinct parties and occur at multiple levels at the same time.
- The healthcare system involves a wide variety of knowledge, power, and control held by the various participants. Although it is normal for most conflicts to involve some level of differences between individuals, what is unusual are the institutionalized differences brought about by differing levels of responsibility and education, as is the case in healthcare (Figure 11-1).
- The ethnic diversity of both consumers and providers of healthcare services in many communities is striking and can create potential barriers to helping participants determine solutions.
- Strong gender inequities remain in healthcare in terms of the services offered to patients, the research done, the opportunities for staff, and the diversity (or lack thereof) within provider groups.
- Healthcare involves people interacting with other people to repair and preserve the health and personal integrity of patients. Often this involves issues about which people may have strongly held personal or religious values that may seem to be, and often are, irreconcilable.

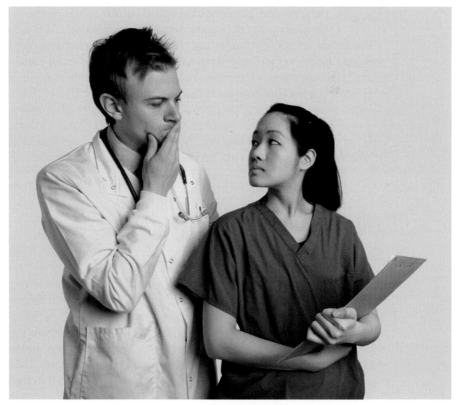

Figure 11-1 The wide variety of knowledge, power, and control held by the various participants in healthcare introduces institutionalized differences in how to handle some situations.

All of these factors combine to make healthcare environments particularly prone to conflict. It is therefore important for healthcare professionals and administrators to understand the origins of conflict and to develop strategies to manage the conflicts they experience.

Discussion
Is a peaceful healthcare environment where all the healthcare providers always get along and avoid conflict always best for the patient?

Positive vs. Negative Conflict

Conflict can appear in a positive, or functional, aspect that can effect improvement as well as a negative, or dysfunctional, aspect that can cause upheaval. **Positive conflict** is the idea that healthy discussion can occur in the face of a disagreement, regardless of different personalities, education levels, or responsibilities. Positive conflict can be utilized in many ways. For example, a competition between hospital departments for the highest patient satisfaction score is positive conflict. Positive conflict can inspire creativity and "thinking outside the box" to resolve a problem. There is a natural tendency to avoid conflict, because it is viewed as hostile and unpleasant. It is important

Relate to Practice
Susan attended a departmental meeting to discuss new attendance policies and clinical guidelines. The discussion became quite heated, separating the department into two factions who argued on both sides of the policy issues. By the end of the meeting, a consensus had been reached and both sides of the issue were satisfied. There was even some good-natured joking between several team members afterward. Later that day during lunch, one of Susan's coworkers started talking about the meeting and how uncomfortable she had been. The coworker stated that she does not like it when people argue and wanted to know why "we all can't just get along." Susan felt the meeting had been exceptionally good and had been glad that everyone's opinions had been heard. What could Susan say to her coworker about conflict?

Relate to Practice
Judy was recently hired as a certified medical assistant in a new pediatrician's office. After working several months, she noticed that another medical assistant, Debbie, was arriving late every day. It was Debbie's job to arrive early to turn on the computers, restock the exam rooms, and make sure the messages from the answering service were given to the physicians. Judy became upset because she not only had to take care of patients but also was left with doing Debbie's job as well. One day Debbie was more than 1 hour late, and the waiting room was packed. Judy muttered under her breath how unfair it was that she was left doing both Debbie's job and her own job. Debbie overheard her. Debbie started to yell at Judy that it was not her fault that traffic was bad.
1. How should Judy handle the situation?
2. What should Debbie do to arrive on time?

to understand that conflict does not have to be a bad or unproductive situation. Although conflict is difficult, it brings growth and change. Conflict can be an indicator that change may be coming or necessary. Negative conflict is when conflict devolves into disruptive behaviors or violence, usually attributable to the lack of trust, communication, and discussion. The important thing to note is that if conflict is identified and managed early, it can lead to a positive result.

Conflict Behavioral Styles

Conflict is often best understood by examining the results of various behaviors. These behaviors are usefully categorized according to conflict styles. Each style is a way to react to a dispute but may impact other people in different ways.

Competing

Competing is a style in which an individual's own needs are advocated over the needs of others. It relies on an aggressive style of communication, low regard for future relationships, and the exercise of coercive power. Those using a competitive style tend to seek control over a discussion. They fear that loss of such control will result in solutions that fail to meet their needs. Competing tends to result in responses that increase the level of threat.

Accommodating

Accommodating, also known as smoothing, is the opposite of competing. People using this style allow the group's needs to take priority over their own in an effort to preserve the relationship.

Avoiding

Avoiding is a common response to the negative perception of conflict. "Give it time, it will blow over," we say to ourselves. But, generally, all that happens is that feelings are repressed, views remain unexpressed, and the conflict festers until it becomes too big to ignore. Like a cancer that may well have been cured if treated early, the conflict grows and spreads until it kills the relationship. Because needs and concerns stay unexpressed, people are often confused, wondering what went wrong in a relationship.

Compromising

Compromising is an approach to conflict in which people gain and give in a series of tradeoffs. Although satisfactory, compromise is generally not satisfying. We each remain entrenched in our individual perceptions and do not necessarily understand the other side very well. We often retain a lack of trust and avoid risk-taking involved in more collaborative behaviors.

Collaborating

Collaborating is the pooling of individual needs and goals toward a common goal. Often called "win-win problem-solving," collaboration requires assertive communication and cooperation in order to achieve the best solution. It offers the chance for agreement, the integration of needs, and the potential to exceed the expectations of the conflict resolution.

Adjustments Based on Behavioral Styles

By understanding each style and its consequences, we may adjust our behaviors in various situations. This does not mean that any one style is better or worse than another, but it does allow us to anticipate and understand the expected consequences of each approach: If we use a competing style, we might force others to accept "our" solution, but this acceptance may be accompanied by fear and resentment. If we accommodate, the relationship may proceed smoothly, but we may foster frustrations that our needs are not being addressed. If we compromise, we may feel fine about the outcome, but still harbor resentments in the future. If we collaborate, we may not gain a better solution than a compromise might have yielded, but we are more likely to feel better about our chances for future understanding and goodwill. And if we avoid discussing the conflict at all, both parties may remain clueless about the real underlying issues and concerns, only to be dealing with them in the future.

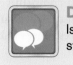

Discussion
Is it possible to have positive conflict with more than one behavior style?

Emotional, Cognitive, and Physical Responses to Conflict

In addition to the behavioral responses summarized by the various conflict styles, we have emotional, cognitive, and physical responses to conflict as well. These are important aspects of our experience during conflict, and they frequently tell us more about what is the true source of our perception of a threat. By understanding our thoughts, feelings, and physical responses to conflict, we may get better insights into the best potential solutions to the situation.

Emotional Responses

These are the feelings we experience in conflict, ranging from anger and fear to despair and confusion. Emotional responses are often misunderstood, because people tend to believe that others feel the same as they do. Thus, differing emotional responses are confusing and, at times, threatening.

Cognitive Responses

These are our ideas and thoughts about a conflict, often present as our inner voice or internal observer in the midst of a situation. For example, we might think any of the following things in response to someone taking a parking spot just as we are ready to park:

"That jerk! Who does he think he is?"
   or
"He sure seems distracted. I wonder if he is okay."
   or

"What am I supposed to do now? I'm going to be late for my meeting. I should give him a piece of my mind! But what if he gets mad at me?"

Such different thoughts contribute to emotional and behavioral responses, where self-talk can promote either a positive or a negative feedback loop in the situation.

Physical Responses

These responses can play an important role in our ability to meet our needs in the conflict. They include heightened stress, physical tension, increased perspiration, tunnel vision, shallow or accelerated breathing, nausea, and rapid heartbeat. These "fight or flight" responses are those we experience in high-anxiety situations, and they may be managed through stress management techniques. Establishing a calmer environment in which emotions can be managed is more likely if the physical response is addressed effectively.

Disruptive Behavior

Disruptive behavior has been defined by the American Medical Association (AMA) as "personal conduct, whether verbal or physical, that affects or that potentially may affect patient care negatively." It specifically includes "conduct that interferes with one's ability to work with other members of the healthcare team." Of course, physicians are not the only individuals who exhibit disruptive behavior, and the challenge is to find a way of addressing any disruptive behavior in healthcare, whether by healthcare workers or by patients. The AMA does not list the behaviors they believe are disruptive. However, it does encourage documentation of the behaviors in a policy with due process safeguards. Even without a list, this step represents a relatively easy structural change that can be managed and controlled to a high degree. The following can be examples of potentially disruptive behaviors among healthcare professionals:

- Profane or disrespectful language
- Demeaning behavior, such as name calling
- Sexual comments or innuendo
- Inappropriate touching, sexual or otherwise
- Racial or ethnic jokes
- Outbursts of anger
- Throwing instruments, charts, or other objects
- Criticizing other caregivers in front of patients or other staff
- Comments that undermine a patient's trust in other caregivers or the hospital
- Failure to adequately address safety concerns or patient care needs expressed by another caregiver
- Intimidating behavior that can suppress input by other members of the healthcare team
- Deliberate failure to adhere to organizational policies without adequate reason
- Retaliation against any member of the healthcare team who has reported an instance of violation of the code of conduct or who has participated in the investigation of such incident, regardless of the perceived veracity of the report

For each item on this list there is an implicit expectation about how healthcare personnel should behave. When behavior is shown that goes against that expectation or if there is the perception that it does, then conflict exists.

Whether it is surgical technologists filing complaints about having instruments thrown at them or medical assistants humiliated by their supervisors, victims of disruptive or abusive behavior may come to view litigation as the only way to protect their safety and dignity. To combat this risk, an increasing number of healthcare organizations are adopting a zero tolerance policy for the most serious offenses (e.g., sexual harassment and physical violence) and offering counseling, education, and training for other offenses. By responding swiftly and decisively to observed incidents or complaints, organizations can protect themselves against liability for condoning a hostile or discriminatory work environment. However, facilities that do not address disruptive and abusive behavior on the part of physicians or staff when it first appears create significant liability exposure for themselves should the behavior recur. In such a situation, it becomes difficult to defend against a claim.

Relate to Practice

A surgical technologist is walking past a scrub sink where he sees a coworker washing her hands and crying. The coworker tells him that during a just-completed procedure the saw stopped working for some reason, and the surgeon "lost it" and threw the saw against the wall while yelling for more equipment. The coworker told him that it upset her to be put into a situation like that, but that she did not know what she could do about it. What could the surgical technologist advise his coworker to do?

Conflict Management

Conflict management is the long-term management of disputes and conflicts, which may or may not lead to resolution. For decades hospitals and other healthcare providers have recognized the need for managing conflict within the healthcare workplace in order to assure that conflict does not affect the quality of care and patient safety.

The **"captain of the ship" doctrine** is an adaptation from the "borrowed servant rules," as applied to an operating room, which arose in *McConnell v. Williams*, placing greatest responsibility on the person in charge (e.g., a surgeon responsible for all under his or her supervision), regardless of whether the "captain" is *directly* responsible for the alleged error or act of alleged negligence, and despite the assistants' positions as hospital employees. While this doctrine was originally interpreted for an operating room setting, over the years it has come to apply to all physician/subordinate interactions, regardless of setting. The old thought process of the physician as "captain of the ship" has yielded to social, regulatory, and legal changes, including gender equality, patient autonomy, and legal accountability/tort liability.

In 2009, **The Joint Commission**, the organization that accredits hospitals and other healthcare organizations, began requiring that healthcare organizations establish policies and procedures for conflict management among leadership groups (Standard LD.02.04.01). The Joint Commission references conflict management in its leadership standards, placing responsibility for implementation and application of conflict management variously on the organization, its governing body, and its leaders. The standards and their elements of performance refer to: (1) "a system for resolving conflicts among individuals working in the hospital" (Standard LD.01.03.01), (2) "an ongoing process for managing conflict among leadership groups" (Standard LD.02.04.01), and (3) "a process for managing disruptive and inappropriate behavior" (Standard LD.03.01.01, Element of Performance 5). It should be noted that The Joint Commission will defer to an organization's good faith judgments and reasonable efforts to meet the conflict management standards. The Joint Commission has also expressed increased concern that disruptive or intimidating behavior can threaten patient safety and quality of care.

In 2008, The Joint Commission issued a Sentinel Event Alert titled *Behaviors That Undermine a Culture of Safety;* it described such behaviors and urged organizations to address unprofessional behaviors through formal policies. The Alert also identified the lack of conflict management skills as a root cause of disruptive behavior. The Joint Commission addressed this by recommending interventions such as educating team members, encouraging interprofessional dialogue, and developing an organizational process for responding to intimidating and disruptive behavior. The important message is that any type of conflict management an organization implemented would be beneficial in creating and maintaining a culture of safety that in turn would promote and protect quality of patient care. The challenge for healthcare organizations is to assess their current problem-solving techniques and responses to conflict. How a particular healthcare organization implements policies and procedures to meet the standards of The Joint Commission will be unique to that organization.

Discussion
Should hospitals/healthcare organizations have punitive disciplinary actions for all disruptive behaviors or just the most serious?

Conflict Resolution

Conflict resolution, the process of ending a disagreement between two or more people in a constructive fashion for all parties involved, is the desired result of conflict management. It is the result of conflict that, if managed properly, can create a positive outcome. Healthcare today uses a team-based approach. Whether the team is an office or department staff, surgical team, or other organization, all healthcare providers are members of interdisciplinary teams.

Interpersonal conflict should be managed and resolved before it degenerates into verbal assault and irreparable damage to a team. Dealing with interpersonal conflict can be a difficult and uncomfortable process. Usually, as team members, we use carefully worded statements to avoid frictions when confronting conflict. So how do we start?

The first step in resolving interpersonal conflict is to acknowledge the existence of the interpersonal conflict. Recognizing the conflict allows team members to build common ground by putting the conflict within the context of the larger goal of the team and the organization. Moreover, the larger goal can help by giving team members a motive for resolving the conflict.

The Rosetta Stone for dealing with conflict is communication. As team members, we all understand the inevitability of interpersonal conflicts. Moreover, as we have established earlier in this chapter, open and supportive communication is vital to a high-performing team. One way to achieve this is by separating the problem from the person. Problems can be debated without damaging working relationships. When interpersonal conflict occurs, all sides of the issue should be recognized without finger-pointing or blaming. Above all, when one team member is yelled at or blamed for something, it has the effect of silencing the whole team. It gives the signal to everyone that dissent is not allowed, and, as we know, dissent is one of the most fertile resources for new ideas.

When faced with conflict, it is natural for team members to become defensive. However defensiveness usually makes it more difficult to resolve a conflict. A conflict-friendly team environment must encourage effective listening. This means listening to one another attentively, without interruption (this includes not having side conversations, doodling, or staring vacantly). The fundamentals to resolving team conflict include the following elements:

1. Before stating one's view, a speaker should seek to understand what others have said. This can be done in a few clarifying sentences.
2. Seek to make explicit what the opposing sides have in common. This helps to reinforce what is shared between the disputants.
3. Whether or not an agreement is reached, team members should thank the other team members for having expressed their views and feelings. Thanking the other recognizes the personal risk the individual took in expressing themselves and should be viewed as an expression of trust and commitment toward the team.

Alternative Dispute Resolution

Conflict does not usually appear instantly as a large dramatic situation; instead it appears in stages. Likewise, so do conflict management and resolution. There are occasions when conflict can progress beyond interpersonal conflict techniques and require a third party to assist with the resolution. **Alternative dispute resolution (ADR)** is the procedure for settling disputes by means other than litigation—such as arbitration, mediation, or mini-trials. ADR procedures are usually less costly and quicker than litigation. They are increasingly being utilized in disputes that would otherwise result in litigation—including labor disputes, divorce actions, and personal injury claims. Many people prefer ADR because they view it as a more creative process focused on problem solving, unlike litigation, which is viewed more as a "win-lose" scenario and can be very adversarial. ADR utilizes the negotiation, mediation, facilitation, and arbitration to resolve conflict.

Negotiation

Negotiation is any communication used in an attempt to achieve a goal, approval, or action by another. Those in allied health use negotiation skills daily when interacting with patients, families, coworkers and employers.

We learn the process of negotiating at a young age. When you were young and asked your parents for four cookies and they said one and you finally settled for two cookies, you were negotiating. Negotiating takes place every time two or more individuals resolve a disagreement, an area of contention, or an area that requires some compromises on one or both sides. It may be formal or informal.

Negotiation is similar to compromising, in that there is a back and forth dialogue with a series of tradeoffs. However, there is a difference between the two. In negotiation, the objective of any negotiation process is to get a win-win result, in which both parties gain or lose together. In the process of compromise one party has to lose something whether the loss is big or small. Always remember one important thing: negotiation can be done without compromise, but compromise cannot be done without negotiation.

Mediation

Mediation is the process by which a neutral third party (an attorney, judge, or other person trained in mediation techniques) facilitates and assists the parties in resolving

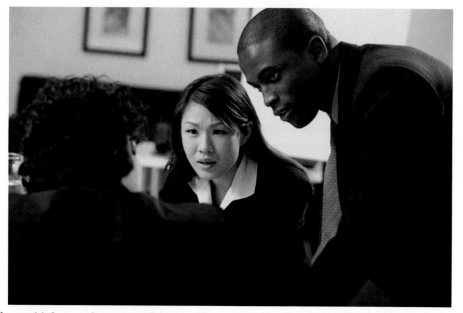

Figure 11-2 A mediator may offer a possible resolution for discussion, help parties explore options, identify issues, and provide information.

a dispute. The fundamental principle of mediation is self-determination. Mediation relies on the ability of the parties to reach a voluntary, uncoerced agreement. The mediator may offer a possible resolution for discussion, help parties explore options, identify issues, and provide information (Figure 11-2).

The mediation process is commonly used to resolve medical malpractice claims, personal injury claims, and employee disputes. It is the least adversarial method of dispute resolution and can assist the individuals to identify the real issues and options for settlement. The individuals maintain control of the outcome.

Facilitation

Facilitation is the process by which a third party (facilitator) assists in the resolution of the dispute. The following are some types of interactive processes that a facilitator may use to resolve issues:

- Guided dialogue
- Consensus building
- Action planning
- Strategic planning
- Vision planning
- Focused conversation
- Systems-change dynamics of human transformation

A trained facilitator uses these processes to guide and aid the group to reach their goals. Every participant is treated as equal and has an impact on the processes used.

Arbitration

Arbitration is the process of resolving issues in conflict in a more structured setting, similar to formal litigation. There can be one arbitrator or a panel of arbitrators that can award damages, interest, attorney's fees, and punitive damages (if allowed by law).

Arbitration is usually voluntary, but the law can mandate it for specific disputes, such as those involving labor and unions.

What If?
A supervisor approaches you and says that a coworker has filed a complaint about your frequent breaks and time spent on the phone. How would you respond? How would you treat that coworker the next time you worked together?

Conclusion

Members of the healthcare team work in stressful environments that can bring about conflict. Conflict is a normal part of human behavior. It may seem unpleasant, but it does have a purpose. Conflict arises when individuals disagree, and then perceive a threat to their needs, interests, or concerns. Conflict drives change, and without it, the world would stagnate. If conflict is managed correctly, it can produce a positive result in which the respective individuals are satisfied with the outcome and change is enacted. The key to successful conflict resolution is communication and honest discussion. If conflict is not addressed, it can devolve into disruptive behavior and lead to litigation. Disruptive behavior not only is harmful to the individuals, but also has been shown to affect patient safety. Healthcare organizations must draft and enact conflict management policies and procedures for the workplace to protect both workers and patients from the harmful effects of negative conflict.

Chapter Review Questions

1. Conflict occurs when one individual perceives a threat to his or her
   A. needs.
   B. interests.
   C. concerns.
   D. All of the above

2. Disruptive behavior is an example of
   A. positive conflict.
   B. negative conflict.
   C. disagreement.
   D. None of the above

3. What is the key point in dealing with conflict to enable a positive outcome?
   A. Communication
   B. Speaking loudly
   C. Waiting to discuss the event
   D. Physical gestures to communicate a point

4. The ADR process that is similar to compromising is
   A. mediation.
   B. arbitration.
   C. negotiation.
   D. facilitation.

5. The conflict behavior style that is also known as "smoothing" is
   A. avoiding.
   B. collaborating.
   C. compromising.
   D. accommodating.

Self-Reflection Questions
1. How do I personally feel about conflict? Why?
2. How would I handle disruptive behavior from a coworker?
3. Is it possible for conflict to be healthy?
4. Does your workplace have a conflict management policy? If so, do you know what it is?
5. Think about a conflict that you have experienced in the past. What was the outcome? Positive or negative? Think about the steps that led to that outcome. Could it have been handled differently?

Internet Activities

1. Go to the website of the International Association for Conflict Management at www. iacm-conflict.com. When were they founded and what is their mission statement?
2. Go to the website of The National Urban Technology Center at www.urbantech.org/ cms/conflictresolution. Why is it important to teach children in K-12 about conflict resolution? What other conflict-related skills do they teach?

Additional Resources

www.healthlawyers.org/hlresources/ADR/Documents/ADRToolkit.pdf
www.rnjournal.com/journal_of_nursing/conflict-resolution-tools-for-nursing.htm
www.jointcommission.org/
www.cspsteam.org
www.ama-assn.org/
www.iacm-conflict.org/

Bibliography

Porto G, Lauve R: Disruptive clinician behavior: a persistent threat to safety, *Patient Safety Quality Healthcare,* July/Aug 2006.
www.healthlawyers.org/hlresources/ADR/Documents/ADRToolkit.pdf
www.rnjournal.com/journal_of_nursing/conflict-resolution-tools-for-nursing.htm
www.cna.com/vcm_content/CNA/internet/Static%20File%20for%20Download/Risk%20Control/ Medical%20Services/DefusingConflictMinimizingRisk.pdf
www.mediate.com/articles/simpson.cfm
www.karlbayer.com/blog/applying-conflict-resolution-skills-in-health-care-part-i-principled -negotiation-method/
http://johnford.blogs.com/jfa/2009/03/contextualizing-disruptive-behavior-in-health-care-as-a- conflict-management-challenge.html
www.ncbi.nlm.nih.gov/pmc/articles/PMC1291328/
www.pon.harvard.edu/category/daily/conflict-management/
www.jointcommission.org/
www.aviationpros.com/article/10385718/conflict-in-the-workplace-conflict-can-be-positive -and-productive
www.ehow.com/about_6802533_description-positive-conflict.html
http://smallbusiness.chron.com/positive-negative-conflicts-workplace-11422.html
http://en.wikibooks.org/wiki/Managing_Groups_and_Teams/Conflict
www.craweblogs.com/commlog/archives/003498.html
http://medical-dictionary.thefreedictionary.com/Captain+of+the+Ship+Doctrine
www.ohrd.wisc.edu/onlinetraining/resolution/aboutwhatisit.htm
Greenhalgh L: Managing conflict, *MIT Sloan Manage Rev* (Summer 2006):45-51, 2006.
Lafasto F, Larson C: *When teams work best,* Thousand Oaks, Calif, 2001, Sage Publications, ISBN 0-7619- 2366-7.
Siegel M: The perils of culture conflict, *Fortune, Nov* 1998:257-262, 1998.
Simons TL, Peterson RS: Task conflict and relationship conflict in top management teams: the pivotal role of intragroup trust, *J Appl Psychol* 85(1):102-111, 2000.
Taylor SM: Manage conflict through negotiation and mediation, *The Blackwell handbook of principles of organizational behavior,* 2003, ISBN 9780631215066.
Weingart L, Jehn KA: Manage intra-team conflict through collaboration, *The Blackwell handbook of principles of organizational behavior,* 2003, ISBN 9780631215066.
http://public.findlaw.com

Chapter 12

Business Aspects of Healthcare

Jeanne McTeigue

KEY TERMS

Associate practice This is a legal agreement in which physicians share staff and overhead expenses of operation but do not share in the legal responsibility or in the profits of business.

CHAMPVA Acronym denoting Civilian Health and Medical Program of the Department of Veterans Affairs. Coverage designed specifically for disabled veterans and their dependents. Also known as Veterans Health Administration.

Co-insurance This is the amount of payment that is agreed upon by the insured as their portion of any claims.

Conscience clause Regulation or mandate stating that healthcare providers and/or facilities do not have to participate in procedures that are against their beliefs, such as abortions or sterilization procedures.

Copay A fixed amount determined by the health insurance policy that is paid for services to offset premiums paid by the insured.

Corporation A company that is established legally and is managed by a board of directors.

Deductible An amount of money that is paid by the insured before the insurance company pays for services. Usually a fixed amount paid annually.

Fee splitting An illegal act of sharing profit or compensation by a physician for referral of patients or incentives for referral of services.

Gatekeeper A person, such as the primary care physician, or an organization that is appointed by an HMO carrier to maintain and approve services to reduce costs and unnecessary spending.

Group practice A medical practice with three or more physicians of the same or similar specialty, who share the same overhead and staff and practice medicine together.

Health Maintenance Organization (HMO) A type of managed care company that serves participating patients by offering services at a fixed rate within the group of participating providers and facilities. A fixed fee schedule is negotiated with the providers as well.

Liability Obligations under law arising from civil actions or torts.

Limited Liability Company (LLC) A legally structured company in which the members of the company cannot be held personally liable for the debts or actions of the company or another party in the company.

Medicaid Federal program administered by each individual state that provides healthcare coverage for the indigent and/or medically needy patients.

Medicare Federal program that provides medical insurance coverage to members older than age 65 or to those who are deemed permanently disabled.

Primary care physician (PCP) A designated provider that oversees the care and manages the healthcare services for an individual.

Professional corporation (PC) A specific legal company structure that is designed for provision of professional services for their clients, such as lawyers, physicians, or architects.

Sole proprietorship A single professional-owned business in which an individual employs other professionals in the same field. In medical practice, a single physician-owned practice that employs other physicians to work for the practice.

Solo practice Single owner/operator of the company or business. In the medical field, this would represent a single physician practice.

Specialist In the medical field, an individual who has undergone further specific training in a certain discipline and practices medicine in that discipline, such as dermatology or endocrinology.

Third party payer Usually refers to an insurance company but can be any other person or organization that is responsible for the medical care coverage of a patient.

TRICARE Government medical program for active duty military and their dependents as well as coverage for military retirees (after 20 or more years of service).

CHAPTER OBJECTIVES

1. Describe types of healthcare providers and professionals.
2. Discuss the rationale for implementing a corporate structure in healthcare practices.
3. Outline the benefits of using mid-level providers.
4. Determine the legality of physician incentives for patient referrals.
5. List and describe types of practice structures.
6. Identify and describe different types of health insurance plans and related patient costs, including HMOs.
7. Describe the different types of government health coverage programs—Medicare, Medicaid, and TRICARE.

Introduction

Most people do not view the practice of medicine as a business, but indeed it is a business and the aspects of its business side will be explored in this chapter. Not every medical practice uses the same type of business structure or model; instead, many factors influence the type of business structure a practice may choose. Some of these factors include the types of patients who are served; changes in reimbursement and billing procedures for providers; and also legal strategies that can offer some protection against personal financial liabilities. This chapter is not meant to recommend a specific business structure, but instead to offer an overview of the various types of healthcare providers and the most common types of business providers, as well as an overview of insurance and government coverage plans.

Types of Providers

We will begin by looking at the various types of healthcare providers so we can understand how they all function together under various corporate structures, such as a health maintenance organization (HMO). Healthcare providers range from physicians and specialists to mid-level providers to allied healthcare professions, such as technicians. All give care to patients. Listed next are specific examples of each of these types of providers.

Medical Doctors

Among physicians, we encounter a wide variety of different degrees and levels of education, including specialized degrees in certain disciplines of medicine. All licensed physicians have undergone a minimum of undergraduate education, and fully completed medical school and internship requirements. Fully licensed physicians may be either medical doctors (MDs) or doctors of osteopathic medicine (DO). Both credentials are equivalent in the practice of medicine; the major difference between the two is the type of medical school that was attended by the physician.

Specialists

These physicians are fully licensed MD or DO medical doctors who have pursued further schooling and training in a specific area of medicine (Figure 12-1). Having completed the additional training and education, they may have the listing of either "board certified" or "fellowship" in those areas, depending on the type of specialty and board that certified the provider. Some of these specialist categories include the following:

- Allergy and immunology
- Anesthesiology
- Cardiology
- Dermatology
- Emergency medicine
- Family practice
- Geriatric medicine
- Hematology
- Infection control
- Internal medicine
- Neurology
- Nephrology

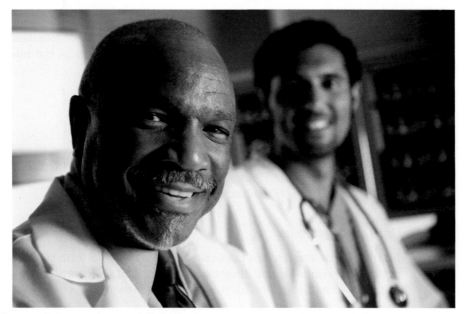

Figure 12-1 Specialists are fully licensed MD or DO medical doctors who have undergone further schooling and training in a specific area of medicine.

- Nuclear medicine
- Obstetrics and gynecology
- Oncology
- Otorhinolaryngology
- Pathology
- Pediatrics
- Physiatry—Physical medicine and rehab
- Preventive medicine
- Psychiatry
- Radiology
- Rheumatology

Surgical specialties include the following:

- General surgery
- Neurosurgery
- Plastic surgery
- Hand surgery
- Colorectal surgery
- Orthopedic surgery
- Oral surgery
- Thoracic surgery

Associations and organizations that these physicians would belong to may include the following:

- AMA—American Medical Association
- American College of Surgeons
- American College of Physicians
- Board specialty organizations in each specialty area

Other Types of Providers

Other areas of allied health–related fields have different requirements for licensure and practice and these vary based on the specific field but are not required to complete the full medical school requirements of an MD or DO. Some of the titles that could be obtained include the following:

- DC—Doctor of Chiropractic
- DMD—Doctor of Dental Medicine
- DDS—Doctor of Dental Surgery
- OD—Doctor of Optometry
- PhD—Doctor of Philosophy (this may be in many different areas, such as psychiatry or engineering)
- DPM—Doctor of Podiatric Medicine

Mid-Level Providers

Mid-level providers are not physicians, but they may perform similar services such as writing prescriptions, and they usually bill insurance companies for their services. Examples of mid-level providers include the following:

- NP—Nurse Practitioner
- PA—Physician's Assistant

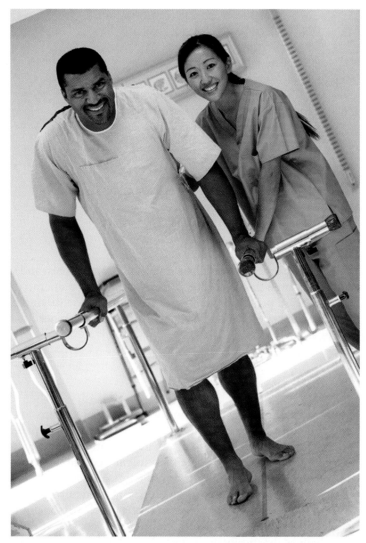

Figure 12-2 Mid-level providers are not physicians, but they may perform similar services such as writing prescriptions, and they usually bill insurance companies for their services. Examples of mid-level providers include physical therapists.

- CRNA—Certified Registered Nurse Anesthetist
- LSW—Licensed Social Worker
- PT—Physical Therapist (Figure 12-2)
- OT—Occupational Therapist

Allied Health Professionals

These individuals are essential members of the healthcare team but instead of billing separately to the insurance carriers for their services, they operate as paid employees, or sometimes as outside contractors paid by the employer or facility. The following list represents only some of the areas of certification and training in the allied health field:

- BSN—Bachelor of Science in Nursing
- CMA/RMA—Certified or Registered Medical Assistant

- CMT—Certified Medical Transcriptionist
- CNA—Certified Nursing Assistant
- CPC—Certified Professional Coder
- Dental Assistant
- Dental Hygienist
- EMT—Emergency Medical Technician
- Laboratory or Medical Technologist
- LPN—Licensed Practical Nurse
- Pharmacist
- Pharmacy Technician
- Phlebotomist
- RHIT—Registered Health Information Technologist
- RN—Registered Nurse
- RT—Respiratory Therapist
- X-Ray Technician

Patients sometimes confuse medical professionals and may, depending on the setting, assume that everyone is either a nurse or a doctor. In facilities like a hospital, all healthcare professionals should have clearly identifying badges or name tags that indicate their specialty and credentials. Students also need to be sure to identify themselves as such.

Corporate Structure

Many years ago, it was commonplace for new physicians to complete medical school, open an office attached to their home, and begin seeing patients, using their personal Social Security number as their tax identification number. However, as the culture of our society changed and the environment became a litigious one, in which patients became inclined to sue physicians, doctors and other providers were losing personal assets and their livelihood in lawsuits. The structuring of the practice as a business then became a way for providers to protect their personal property and assets in cases of a lawsuit. By the 1980s, health maintenance organizations (HMOs) became popular and changed drastically the system of reimbursement for providers. Therefore it became necessary for many professionals to unify to share costs and overhead expenses in order to remain profitable.

For all these reasons and others, the number of providers working in solo practice has diminished because it has become necessary to work in groups using a corporate structure. Besides protection of assets, incorporation has brought many other positive benefits. For example, working in a corporate group gives the providers another partner or provider who can handle their patients easily if they are not available. Before the utilization of this structure, a physician was, by necessity, always "on call." Taking a day of vacation, for example, necessitated asking another physician solo practice to cover for the physician. By contrast, the benefit for both the patient and the covering physician in a group or multiple-doctor practice is that the covering physician can access all of the clinics' medical records and may even already be familiar with the patient in question. It is also a benefit to the provider who is unavailable, making it easier to take a day of vacation as well as causing less worry about their patients' management.

Another challenge in a solo practice occurred when a physician passed away. Unless the spouse was also a physician, the surviving spouse and/or dependents were not able to continue the practice or inherit the profits of the practice. Many widowed spouses in these instances would have to "sell" the practice to another provider, who would then assume the care of those patients. In a corporate structure, the assets could be distributed and willed to surviving family and a negotiated share of the corporation could be inherited. This also meant the estate would not have to "sell" the practice; it would just be taken over by the remaining physicians or providers.

Using Mid-Level Providers

In addition to adopting a more corporate structure, practices now commonly employ "mid-level providers" such as physician assistants (PAs) or nurse practitioners (NPs), who can assist in seeing patients and handling emergencies. These individuals' roles have been greatly expanded in recent years. Originally, these mid-level providers worked only under the direct supervision of a physician and their services were billed to the insurances and third party payers as if the physician had seen the patient. Guidelines specified that the physician had to be in the office while the mid-level provider was seeing patients in case there was a problem or a question. In addition, they were only utilized for seeing overflow patients and routine follow-up care without any complicating factors. Now, however, the role of mid-level providers has changed dramatically so that almost all third party payers recognize their services separately and their services are billable under the credentials of the mid-level provider directly. Some mid-level providers, such as nurse practitioners (NPs), can even open their own practices. Their expertise has increased such that they no longer have to be under the direct supervision of the physician. The majority of insurance carriers, however, do reduce the amount of reimbursement for services provided by a mid-level provider instead of a physician.

Fee Splitting

It is important to understand that under the law, physicians cannot give incentives for referral of patients to their practices or for referral of services. Fee splitting is an illegal act of sharing profit or compensation by a physician for referral of patients or incentives for referral of services.

The STARK laws (discussed in previous chapters) were designed to protect patients from unnecessary or unethical practices for financial gain. If a physician were to offer reduced fees for patient services based on referral of other patients or if they were to

What If?

? A patient sees an attorney for representation in a workers' compensation case. The attorney, John Jones, recommends that the patient see Dr. Smith, an orthopedic surgeon. The patient is seen by the physician. Then, the next week the physician sends the attorney tickets to the next local professional basketball game because he knows that Mr. Jones likes that team and he wants to thank him for the referral.

1. Is this legal?
2. Is this ethical?
3. How could the patients suffer from these types of situations?

Discussion

Read the following scenarios and determine if they are legal or illegal:

1. A pharmaceutical representative gives a physician a golfing trip as a thank-you for using their new drug that was just released to the market.
2. A physician has a contest for patient referrals to win a gift basket.
3. A local pharmacy always uses the same durable medical equipment vendor because it is owned by the local orthopedic physician who sends all his patients to them.
4. A local group practice purchases a radiology facility in the neighborhood and advertises their purchase in their waiting room and at the radiology facility indicating their new ownership of it.

offer an incentive to an area lawyer or other professional for referral of patients, as an example, these actions would be illegal. If a provider has a vested interest in another healthcare-related business, it must be clearly disclosed by signs or notifications so that patients are aware and realize that they do not have to use that facility. For example, if a physician owns a pharmacy down the street and would profit from his patients using that pharmacy, he or she cannot refer patients to that business without making them fully aware that they are financially connected to that business and the physician can suggest other competing businesses to the patient instead.

Types of Practice Structures

The following examples are meant to provide a general understanding of how practices can be structured, but the listing is not intended to be all-inclusive. There are many different types of corporate structures and even many different variations within those structures, so it would be difficult to represent all the variations.

Solo Practice

In this type of practice, a single physician is the only provider within that practice and does not share patients with any other physicians. In this type of business arrangement, a "covering physician" is necessary when the physician either is away or unable to see patients. Most physicians in solo practice are specialists (although there are some general medicine physicians who work alone as well), and most solo practices are structured as a **PC** or "**professional corporation.**" One of the advantages of this structure is the ability to run the practice without question from a partner or associate. This helps ease operations that would normally fall under the **conscience clause**, which is a mandate that states that healthcare providers and/or facilities do not have to participate in procedures that are against their beliefs, such as abortions or sterilization procedures. In a **group practice**, responses to these kinds of issues would have to be discussed and reach consensus as a group.

Sole Proprietorship

The structure of the **sole proprietorship** is similar to that of the solo practice except that, in this case, the provider has legal agreements to hire other physicians or

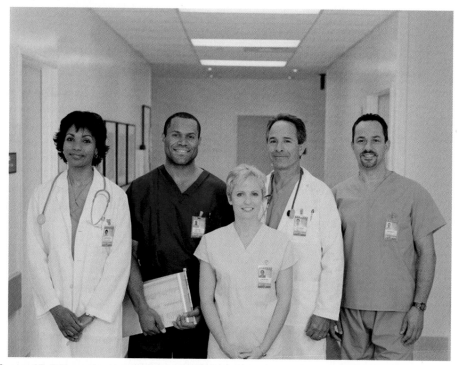

Figure 12-3 In a sole proprietorship, the provider has legal agreements to hire other physicians or mid-level providers to work for them.

mid-level providers to work for them (Figure 12-3). A single physician still owns the practice and employs other providers to work on an hourly or daily basis. In turn, of course, the other providers do not usually share in corporate profits.

Associate Practice

An associate practice is a common structure in which two or more providers (usually in the same or similar specialty) share the same office staff and space with shared overhead expenses but do not share in the profits, losses, or liabilities of the other physicians' practice. Only the overhead is shared in these cases. These corporate structures can be organized as individual PCs (professional corporations) or could be established as LLCs (limited liability companies).

Group Practice

Although they can involve many variations in size, compensation structure, and profit sharing, what group practices have in common is a corporate structure that assigns designated officers to manage the group, not only enabling the individual physicians to be covered when they are unable to see patients but also enabling them to share overhead and staffing costs and personal protection from liability. Many corporate groups purchase and own their own buildings, which affords the corporation the ability to limit their own costs and, in some cases, even collect rent from other allied health or physicians who rent space from them. The group structure usually provides designed profit sharing and incentives for physicians working together and offers benefits to each provider depending on the level of provider and the length of time associated with the group. This has become one of the most common structures because it benefits and protects the individual physicians/providers.

Other Structures

Some physicians or providers prefer to simply be hired by a hospital directly or by an HMO or staffing type of facility. In all three examples, the providers are direct employees and receive wages, as well as other possible benefits such as liability insurance, as per their contracted agreements, but do not benefit from any profit sharing. Many hospitals are structured this way for hiring of staff physicians, possibly emergency department physicians, radiologists, and anesthesiologists. In any case, the providers have no ownership of the practice or organization; thus, as employees, when leaving work, they would not have to provide coverage for themselves because the facility would be responsible for the coverage of the provider.

Types of Insurance Coverage

Commercial Patient Plans

Point-of-Service Health Insurance

The types of insurance coverage for patients can be confusing. It is not the intention to present here every type of insurance coverage possible but to give an overview of the different types of plans available to patients and to describe patients who are eligible to have these insurance coverages.

Plans vary widely with regard to the patient's liability or the patient's responsibility for payment. If the patient has a **deductible**, this amount would have to be paid first before the insurance carrier would cover any of the claims.

Some patients have a larger deductible in order to save on the monthly premiums for the coverage. This works well for patients who are rarely sick, take few medications, and mainly need health insurance to cover them in emergency situations or in cases of catastrophic illness. Some employers carry this type of plan for their employees as well because it is less expensive for them if they are paying part or all of the monthly premiums for their employees. The employer may offer a Health Savings Plan or another similar option for employees to use to offset the high deductible.

Some plans have a copay that a patient must pay at time of service, with the insurance carrier paying a percentage and the patient paying the remainder of the bill. For instance, if a patient has an 80/20 plan, this means that the insurance carrier is paying 80% of the fees and the patient is responsible for 20%. This is called a point-of-service plan. In this type of plan, the physician or provider cooperates with the insurance company by accepting an adjusted fee scale. In other words, under the terms of the agreement, fees are based on what the insurance company allows for the service, and not on what is billed by the physician.

Refer to Box 12-1. Suppose Megan, a patient with health insurance, visits Dr. X, who accepts her particular insurance. Dr. X's fee is normally $120 for an office visit, but because he accepts Megan's insurance plan, he charges only $80—an amount dictated by the insurance plan. Megan's policy states that the company pays 80%, whereas Megan is responsible for the remaining 20%. Eighty percent of $80 is $64. Thus, the insurance company pays $64, and Megan is responsible for the remaining $16.

This means that *the service itself* would cost a lot more for a patient paying out-of-pocket than it does if the physician is participating with the patient's insurance plan and is willing to accept the insurance company's fee schedule. In the example of our

BOX 12-1
Megan's Office Visit Is Covered

Dr. X participates with insurance:
    Office visit: $120
    Insurance allows: $80
    Insurance pays 80%: $64
    Patient has co-insurance at 20%: $16

BOX 12-2
Megan's Office Visit—Without Health Insurance

Dr. X does NOT participate with insurance:
    Office visit: $120
    Patient pays: $120

BOX 12-3
Megan's Office Visit—Insurance Allows Reimbursement

Dr. X does not participate with insurance:
Office visit: $120
Insurance allows $80 in reimbursement only, not at point-of-service
Insurance pays 80%: $64
Patient pays: $120; submits and awaits reimbursement of $80 (eventually
    paying $40 total out-of-pocket after reimbursement)

patient Megan, the same office visit without insurance will be billed to Megan at $120 (see Box 12-2).

Now suppose that the patient still wants to use a physician who rejects her insurance plan's reduced fee. In some plans, she would have to pay out-of-pocket—at a cost of $120 for that office visit, as we see in Box 12-2. But sometimes an insurance plan allows the patient to choose the physician of her choice, regardless of whether the physician is in their plan. So how does that work? It means that the insurance company is willing to pay its standard $80, and since the physician will not accept that fee, Megan may still use this doctor but *now she must pay the difference between the $80 and the $120.* Thus, she will pay $40 of the $120 fee—instead of paying $16 out of the $80 fee. Usually, in this arrangement, since the physician rejects the plan, Megan must pay the $120 in full at the point of service, and then file the bill with her plan and petition to receive $80 back from the insurance company (Box 12-3). *However, this is not available with all insurance plans.*

Health Maintenance Organizations
If the patient has an HMO or health maintenance organization type plan (sometimes called a managed care plan), then there is no co-insurance amount due but instead a flat copayment fee for the services provided. In the case of a managed care plan, the patient may have a $5, $10, $20 copay depending on the plan, but it will be a set amount due at the time of service. Some of these plans have different copays due for prescriptions or hospital services, but in all cases their copayment amount will be a set flat fee.

HMOs or managed care plans became popular in the 1980s. Today the majority of local healthcare plans are some type of managed care plan. The disadvantage of HMO plans is when, in a strict HMO, the insured can only see the participating providers in that plan. In cases of a strict HMO, the patient has to have a PCP, or primary care physician, who manages his or her health and gives referrals for any specialists needed for consultation.

In the HMO models, the focus is on preventive medicine, and the PCP is the gate-keeper who oversees and gives the patient continuity of care, instead of having the patient see a number of different doctors. This centralized approach helps to reduce the possibility of unnecessary testing that can occur when communication among multiple providers worsens. Instead, the PCP can access and manage the patient's health from a more unified, overall vantage point. In the past, the problem with this model initially was that a provider could be financially penalized by the HMO if too many referrals were given in a month. This played at odds with a physician's duty. It is important that providers always keep the medical necessity of the patient foremost. If it is medically necessary for the patient, then the physician is ethically bound to treat (or refer) the patient first. For this important reason, the policy of financially penalizing HMO providers has been discontinued.

A second problem with the original HMO plans was that in some cases some of the employees did not have access to the participating providers that were listed. Also, if the patient wanted to see a physician who was not in the network, they would have to pay for those services completely on their own (remember Megan's dilemma in Box 12-2). This challenge inspired the development of the EPO (exclusive provider organization) or PPO (preferred provider organization). Under this plan, if the patient sees a provider who does participate with the plan then the patient pays the flat copay amount (as in Box 12-1). If the patient chooses to see a provider who does not participate with the plan, the patient can still see the provider but the patient must pay up front and then be reimbursed based on the percentage (out of network) benefit of 80/20 or 70/30, for example, and maybe a deductible as well. These types of plans are very popular and are generally the most common plans seen through large employers.

Other Commercial Payers

Other types of commercial plans include self-insured models, in which the employer establishes a savings account and provides funds to that account to cover employees' claims; this is called an ERISA type plan. Others use a combination: they implement the self-insured model up to a set amount and then the insurance carrier pays above and beyond that amount.

Most car accidental injury policies are covered like a commercial carrier, and generally most insured individuals will have some type of deductible associated with their plans; this is billed to the individual's *"no fault"* car insurance carrier. In most cases each party deals with their own insurance plan for medical coverage and then, if needed, one party in the accident may sometimes be taken to court over any necessary settlements.

Workers' Compensation

Workers' compensation plans are generally handled like a commercial payer but involve some additional, specialized steps such as reporting a new disability and applying to the employer and the employer's insurance carrier for either coverage or reimbursement of a percentage of the damages done.

Any third party payer would be considered commercial. For example, a patient is injured while shopping and the retail store is covering the expenses, or Person A is injured on the front steps of Person B's home and wants Person B's insurance to cover expenses. Either case will require a "third party" payer, which refers to the insurance carrier for the liable party for the injury.

Government Carriers

Medicaid

Medicaid is a federal program that is governed and managed by each individual state to give aid to the indigent or medically needy patient. Many times the department of social services for the area will manage who is eligible for coverage and any other benefits that might be awarded to an individual. Often when a patient is not financially needy, they may be considered medically needy because of a catastrophic illness or injury. Also, in many states, special programs are in place for needy children and pregnant women to ensure that they are also covered as needed. Most of the regular programs are free, but the child coverage in most states may have a minimal premium that the parents might have to contribute. Although these are federally funded programs, each individual state regulates the programs so the conditions, eligibility requirements, and benefits vary among states. Also, until recently, there were a few states that did not offer these plans, but now all 50 states have programs.

On the state distribution level, these programs usually use local HMO carriers to administer and manage eligible patients, and these eligible patients choose from a selection of these HMOs, giving the Medicaid recipient more choices when looking for providers.

Medicare

Medicare is a federal program for coverage of eligible recipients age 65 or older. Generally these recipients become eligible at age 65 to apply for Social Security benefits at the same time. This coverage is also given to permanently disabled individuals as well. Individuals who become permanently disabled and unable to work may apply for Medicare coverage after 24 months of permanent disability. This waiting period of 24 months is reduced in cases of ESRD (end-stage renal disease) to 2 months. This coverage is also available to permanently disabled children.

There are three parts to Medicare:

- Medicare part A: Covers hospital claims
- Medicare part B: Covers all outpatient services
- Medicare part D: Covers the prescription drug plan

Medicare part C is for the eligible Medicare recipient who opts to be covered by an HMO type of Medicare plan. As with Medicaid, Medicare offers local participating physicians and generally operates the same as an HMO plan by making patients responsible for a flat copay amount instead of the 80/20 coverage of regular Medicare. Medicare also has a deductible for each part, and usually Medicare recipients need to carry a secondary insurance to cover those co-insurance amounts, or a patient may have Medicare and Medicaid if he or she is medically or financially eligible. The latter is sometimes referred to as "Medi-Medi" plan.

TRICARE

TRICARE (formerly known as the Civilian Health and Medical Program of the Uniformed Services, or CHAMPUS) coverage refers to the plans that cover active military individuals and their dependents, as well as retired military personnel who have served for 20 years or more. The TRICARE program is managed by the Tricare Management Activity (TMA) under the authority of the Assistant Secretary of Defense (Health

Affairs). Enlisted persons who only serve a few years are not eligible for TRICARE once they leave their branch of service but may be eligible for other veterans' benefits. CHAMPVA (Civilian Health and Medical Program of the Department of Veterans Affairs, or Veterans Health Administration) is coverage designed specifically for disabled veterans and their dependents. CHAMPVA (or Veterans Health Administration) is a component of the U.S. Department of Veterans Affairs (VA) and is led by the Under Secretary of Veterans Affairs for Health.

Conclusion

Over the years many aspects of the healthcare field have advanced and changed; and the types of providers of care, the types of services rendered, and the insurance carriers available to cover them have all advanced as well. As we move forward in the years to come, many more changes will be arising in the healthcare field in these areas. Always moving forward and using the newest technologies to care for and cure patients is the most important focus. Healthcare coverage for all persons is an admirable goal toward improving lives everywhere.

Chapter Review Questions

1. What type of practice structure would include a physician who hires other physicians?
   A. Solo practice
   B. Group practice
   C. Sole proprietorship
   D. All the above

2. What type of insurance covers patients who are indigent?
   A. Medicare
   B. Medicaid
   C. Tricare
   D. HMO

3. What type of provider would have the initials DC after his or her name?
   A. Podiatrist
   B. Pharmacist
   C. Chiropractor
   D. None of the above

4. What is an example of a gatekeeper?
   A. An employer
   B. A PCP
   C. A mid-level provider
   D. None of the above

5. What is the mandate that allows individuals to refuse to perform or participate in a treatment or procedure that is against their beliefs?
   A. Good Samaritan laws
   B. *Respondeat superior*
   C. Conscience clause
   D. They cannot refuse

Self-Reflection Questions
1. What areas of concern are there as we move forward with a government health plan?
2. What ethical concerns can be affected by the conscience clause?
3. In what type of practice structure would be most beneficial for you to participate?
4. How do the different types of insurance coverage affect a patient's treatment?

Internet Activities

1. Investigate this and other sites to find out details and facts about ObamaCare: www.obamacarefacts.com.
2. Find out the details of who is eligible for Medicaid in your state and also the eligibility requirements. See www.cms.gov.
3. Investigate the conscience clause and see details of how this developed. Visit www.americanbar.org.

Additional Resources

http://get.empireblue.com
www.cms.gov
www.ama.com
www.americanbar.org
www.bioethics.net
www.tricare.gov

Appendix A

Resource Section

Academy of Nutrition and Dietetics
120 S. Riverside Plaza, Suite 2000
Chicago, IL 60606
Phone: (312) 899-0040
www.eatright.org

Alliance of Cardiovascular Professionals
P.O. Box 2007
Midlothian, VA 23113
Phone: (804) 632-0078
Fax: (804) 639-9212
www.acp-online.org

American Academy of Anesthesiologist Assistants
2209 Dickens Rd.
Richmond, VA 23230
Phone: (804) 565-6353
Fax: (804) 282-0090
www.anesthetist.org

American Academy of Physician Assistants
2318 Mill Rd., Suite 1300
Alexandria, VA 22314
Phone: (703) 836-2272
Fax: (703) 684-1924
www.aapa.org

American Academy of Professional Coders
2480 S. 3850 West, Suite B
Salt Lake City, UT 84120
Phone: (801) 236-2200
Fax: (801) 236-2258
www.aapc.com

American Art Therapy Association
4875 Eisenhower Ave., Suite 240
Alexandria, VA 22304
Phone: (703) 548-5860
Fax: (703) 783-8468
www.arttherapy.org

American Association for Respiratory Care
9425 N. MacArthur Blvd., Suite 100
Irving, TX 75063
Phone: (972) 243-2272
Fax: (972) 484-2720
www.aarc.org

American Association of Blood Banks
8101 Glenbrook Rd.
Bethesda, MD 20814
Phone: (301) 907-6977
Fax: (301) 907-6895
www.aabb.org

American Association of Cardiovascular and Pulmonary Rehabilitation
330 N. Wabash Ave., Suite 2000
Chicago, IL 60611
Phone: (312) 321-5146
Fax: (312) 673-6924
www.aacvpr.org

American Association of Colleges of Pharmacy
1727 King St.
Alexandria, VA 22314
Phone: (703) 739-2330
Fax: (703) 836-8982
www.aacp.org

American Association of Dental Maxillofacial Radiographic Technicians
www.aadmrt.com

American Association of Healthcare Administrative Management
11240 Waples Mill Rd., Suite 200
Fairfax, VA 22030
Phone: (703) 281-4043
Fax: (703) 359-7562
www.aaham.org

American Association of Medical Assistants
20 N. Wacker Dr., Suite 1575
Chicago, IL 60606
Phone: (312) 899-1500
Fax: (312) 899-1259
www.aama-ntl.org

American Association of Medical Dosimetrists
2201 Cooperative Way, Suite 600
Herndon, VA 20171
Phone: (703) 677-8071
Fax: (703) 677-8071
www.medicaldosimetry.com

American Association of Pathologists' Assistants
2345 Rice St., Suite 220
St. Paul, MN 55113
Phone: (651) 697-9264
Fax: (651) 317-8048
www.pathologistsassistants.org

American Association of Pharmacy Technicians
P.O. Box 1447
Greensboro, NC 27402
Phone: (336) 333-9356
Fax: (336) 333-9068
www.pharmacytechnician.com

American Chiropractic Association
1701 Clarendon Blvd.
Arlington, VA 22209
Phone: (703) 276-8800
Fax: (703) 243-2593
www.acatoday.org

American College of Sports Medicine
401 W. Michigan St.
Indianapolis, IN 46202
Phone: (317) 637-9200
Fax: (317) 634-7817
www.acsm.org

American Dental Assistants Association
35 E. Wacker Dr., Suite 1730
Chicago, IL 60601
Phone: (312) 541-1550
Fax: (312) 541-1496
www.dentalassistant.org

American Dental Hygienists' Association
444 N. Michigan Ave., Suite 3400
Chicago, IL 60611
Phone: (312) 440-8900
www.adha.org

American Health Information Management Association
233 N. Michigan Ave., 21st Floor
Chicago, IL 60601
Phone: (312) 233-1100
Fax: (312) 233-1090
www.ahima.org

American Kinesiotherapy Association
118 College Dr., #5142
Hattiesburg, MS 39406
Phone: (800) 296-2582
www.akta.org

American Massage Therapy Association
500 Davis St., Suite 900
Evanston, IL 60201
Phone: (847) 864-0123
Fax: (847) 864-5196
www.amtamassage.org

American Medical Technologists
10700 W. Higgins Rd., Suite 150
Rosemont, IL 60018
Phone: (847) 823-5169
Fax: (847) 823-0458
www.americanmedtech.org

American Music Therapy Association
8455 Colesville Rd., Suite 1000
Silver Spring, MD 20910
Phone: (301) 589-3300
Fax: (301) 589-5175
www.musictherapy.org

American Occupational Therapy Association
4720 Montgomery Lane, Suite 200
Bethesda, MD 20814
Phone: (301) 652-6611
Fax: (301) 652-7711
www.aota.org

American Optometric Association
243 N. Lindbergh Blvd., Floor 1
St. Louis, MO 63141
Phone: (800) 365-2219
www.aoa.org

American Orthoptic Council
3914 Nakoma Rd.
Madison, WI 53711
Phone: (608) 233-5383
Fax: (608) 263-4247
www.orthoptics.org

American Pharmacists Association
2215 Constitution Ave. NW
Washington, DC 20037
Phone: (202) 628-4410
Fax: (202) 783-2351
www.pharmacist.com

American Physical Therapy Association
1111 N. Fairfax St.
Alexandria, VA 22314
Phone: (703) 684-2782
Fax: (703) 684-7343
www.apta.org

**American Society for Clinical Laboratory
Science**
1861 International Dr., Suite 200
McLean, VA 22102
Phone: (571) 748-3770
www.ascls.org

American Society for Clinical Pathology
33 W. Monroe St., Suite 1600
Chicago, IL 60603
Phone: (312) 541-4999
Fax: (312) 541-4998
www.ascp.org

**American Society for Healthcare Risk
Management**
155 N. Wacker Dr., Suite 400
Chicago, IL 60606
Phone: (312) 422-3980
Fax: (312) 422-4580
www.ashrm.org

**American Society of Anesthesia
Technologists and Technicians**
7044 S. 13th St.
Oak Creek, WI 53154
Phone: (414) 908-4942, ext. 450
Fax: (414) 768-8001
www.asatt.org

American Society of Cytopathology
100 W. 10th St., Suite 605
Wilmington, DE 19801
Phone: (302) 543-6583
Fax: (302) 543-6597
www.cytopathology.org

American Society of Echocardiography
2100 Gateway Centre Blvd., Suite 310
Morrisville, NC 27560
Phone: (919) 861-5574
Fax: (919) 882-9900
www.asecho.org

**American Society of Extracorporeal
Technologists**
2209 Dickens Rd.
Richmond, VA 23230
Phone: (804) 565-6363
Fax: (804) 282-0090
www.amsect.org

**American Society of Health-System
Pharmacists**
7272 Wisconsin Ave.
Bethesda, MD 20814
Phone: (866) 279-0681
www.ashp.org

**American Society of Radiologic
Technologists**
15000 Central Ave. SE
Albuquerque, NM 87123
Phone: (800) 444-2778
Fax: (505) 298-5063
www.asrt.org

**American Speech-Language-Hearing
Association**
2200 Research Blvd.
Rockville, MD 20850
Phone: (301) 296-5700
www.asha.org

**Association for Healthcare Administrative
Professionals**
455 S. Fourth St., Suite 650
Louisville, KY 40202
Phone: (502) 574-9040
Fax: (502) 589-3602
www.ahcap.org

Association for Healthcare Documentation Integrity
4230 Kiernan Ave., Suite 170
Modesto, CA 95356
Phone: (209) 527-9620
Fax: (209) 527-9633
www.ahdionline.org

Association for Professionals in Infection Control and Epidemiology
1275 K St., NW, Suite 1000
Washington, DC 20005
Phone: (202) 789-1890
Fax: (202) 789-1899
www.apic.org

Association of Surgical Technologists
6 W. Dry Creek Circle, Suite 20
Littleton, CO 80120
Phone: (303) 694-9130
Fax: (303) 694-9169
www.ast.org

Association of Vascular and Interventional Radiographers
2201 Cooperative Way, Suite 600
Herndon, VA 20171
Phone: (571) 252-7174
www.avir.org

Clinical Exercise Physiology Association
401 W. Michigan St.
Indianapolis, IN 46202
Phone: (317) 637-9200, ext. 148
www.acsm-cepa.org

Clinical Laboratory Management Association
330 N. Wabash Ave., Suite 2000
Chicago, IL 60611
Phone: (312) 321-5111
www.clma.org

Federation of State Boards of Physical Therapy
124 West St. South, Third Floor
Alexandria, VA 22314
Phone: (703) 299-3100
Fax: (703) 299-3110
www.fsbpt.org

International Society for Clinical Densitometry
306 Industrial Park Rd., Suite 208
Middletown, CT 06457
Phone: (860) 259-1000
Fax: (860) 259-1030
www.iscd.org

National Association Medical Staff Services
2025 M St. NW
Washington, DC 20036
Phone: (202) 367-1196
Fax: (202) 367-2196
www.namss.org

National Association of Boards of Pharmacy
1600 Feehanville Dr.
Mount Prospect, IL 60056
Phone: (847) 391-4406
Fax: (847) 391-4502
www.nabp.net

National Association of Dental Laboratories
325 John Knox Rd., #L103
Tallahassee, FL 32303
Phone: (800) 950-1150
Fax: (850) 222-0053
www.nadl.org

National Association of Emergency Medical Technicians
132-A E. Northside Dr.
Clinton, MS 39056
Phone: (601) 924-7744
Fax: (601) 924-7325
www.naemt.org

National Association of Health Care Assistants
501 E. 15th St.
Joplin, MO 64804
Phone: (417) 623-6049
Fax: (417) 623-2230
www.nahcacares.org

National Athletic Trainers' Association
2952 Stemmons Freeway #200
Dallas, TX 75247
Phone: (214) 637-6282
Fax: (214) 637-2206
www.nata.org

National Board for Respiratory Care
18000 W. 105th St.
Olathe, KS 66061
Phone: (913) 895-4900
Fax: (913) 895-4650
www.nbrc.org

National Community Pharmacists Association
100 Daingerfield Rd.
Alexandria, VA 22314
Phone: (703) 683-8200
Fax: (703) 683-3619
www.ncpanet.org

National Dental Hygienists' Association
www.ndhaonline.org

National Health and Exercise Science Association
3701 Flintridge Court
Brookeville, MD 20833
Phone: (301) 576-0611
Fax: (301) 685-1819
www.nhesa.org

National Healthcareer Association
11161 Overbrook Rd.
Leawood, KS 66211
Phone: (800) 499-9092
Fax: (913) 661-6291
www.nhanow.com

National Network of Career Nursing Assistants
3577 Easton Rd.
Norton, OH 44203
Phone: (330) 825-9342
Fax: (330) 825-9378
www.cna-network.org

National Pharmacy Technician Association
P.O. Box 683148
Houston, TX 77268
Phone: (888) 247-8700
Fax: (888) 247-8706
www.pharmacytechnician.org

National Rehabilitation Association
P.O. Box 150235
Alexandria, VA 22315
Phone: (703) 836-0850
Fax: (703) 836-0848
www.nationalrehab.org

National Society for Histotechnology
8850 Stanford Blvd., Suite 2900
Columbia, MD 21045
Phone: (443) 535-4060
Fax: (443) 535-4055
www.nsh.org

National Surgical Assistant Association
1425 K St. NW, Suite 350
Washington, DC 20005
Phone: (202) 266-9951
Fax: (202) 587-5610
www.nsaa.net

Professional Association of Healthcare Coding Specialists
218 E. Bearss Ave., #354
Tampa, FL 33613
Phone: (888) 708-4707
Fax: (813) 333-1596
www.pahcs.org

Society for Vascular Ultrasound
4601 Presidents Dr., Suite 260
Lanham, MD 20706
Phone: (301) 459-7550
Fax: (301) 459-5651
www.svunet.org

Society of Diagnostic Medical Sonography
2745 Dallas Pkwy., Suite 350
Plano, TX 75093
Phone: (214) 473-8057
Fax: (214) 473-8563
www.sdms.org

The Trial Process

1. Prelitigation medical review panel or tribunal (does not apply in all states for medical malpractice claims)
2. Filing of the lawsuit in the appropriate state or federal court
3. Discovery: various techniques (e.g., depositions, interrogatories, requests for production of documents, admissions of pertinent information relating to the facts and issues of the case)
4. Pretrial settlement hearing
5. Mediation before trial
6. Trial by judge or jury
7. Appeal of the decision or judgment

Case Discussions

Case Discussion 1: Altercation with Patient

A certified nursing assistant was involved in an altercation with an Alzheimer's patient; the patient suffered injuries including hematomas near the eyebrows, a skin tear on her forearm, and bruises to the face and neck and around the eyes. The trial court rendered a judgment against the medical center for $40,000 and against the nursing assistant for $25,000. The Tennessee Court of Appeals at Nashville affirmed the trial court's decision against the nursing assistant and reversed the judgment against the medical center because the Government Tort Liability Act does not permit the plaintiff to sue the medical center for the nursing assistant's intentional tort. (The plaintiff's claim was based on the legal doctrines of negligent retention or vicarious liability. A claim for negligent retention was based on the plaintiff's claim that the medical center had prior notice of the nursing assistant's propensity for violence on the basis of an earlier incident.) The Supreme Court of Tennessee held that the harm arising from the intentional acts of the nursing assistant was a forseeable risk created by the negligent medical center. The Court held that each tortfeasor part was jointly and severally liable for the entire amount of damages awarded. The Court reversed in part and affirmed in part the Court of Appeals and remanded the case to the Circuit Court to determine the total amount of damages to be awarded to the plaintiff.[1]

Case Discussion 2: Student Terminated from Program

In *Kimberg*[2] the plaintiff entered the School of Nurse Anesthesia as a graduate student. The plaintiff argued that his payment of tuition, acceptance into the program, and matriculation created an implied-in-fact contract that required the school to comply with the student handbook. He alleged his termination violated rules and regulations for students in the program, the clinical grading policy, and daily verbal and written evaluations and procedures. The defendant alleged the plaintiff refused to communicate with regard to a demonstration that was to be performed on a mannequin and that he was placed on probation even though he had 12 positive clinical evaluations. He was terminated from the program for failing to progress during an alleged probationary period. The court:

---

[1] *Limbaugh v. Coffee Medical Center,* 59 S.W. 73 (Tenn. 10/16/2001).
[2] *Kimberg v. Univ. of Scranton,* No. 3:06cv1209 (M.D. Pa filed Feb 2, 2007).

1. Denied the defendant's motion for dismissal with respect to the breach of contract claim.
2. Granted a motion for dismissal with regard to the claim for breach of covenant of good faith and fair dealing.
3. Held that due process claim issues must be addressed at trial or in a motion for summary judgment with regard to whether the parties complied with the procedural requirements and the policy of not allowing an attorney present during the hearing was not fundamentally unfair.
4. Dismissed the plaintiff's claims for tortuous interference with a contract claim and for punitive damages.

Case Discussion 3: Notification of Abnormality in X-Ray

In *Stanley*[1] a radiologist evaluated a chest x-ray of a nurse as part of a preemployment tuberculosis screening. His report stated the x-ray showed abnormalities including "a small nodule overlying the right sixth rib." A company policy required the prospective employer to notify the nurse (prospective employee) of the results within 72 hours, which was not done. Ten months later she was diagnosed with lung cancer.

Did the radiologist evaluating a chest x-ray for a preemployment tuberculosis screening owe a duty of care to the prospective employee nurse to inform her or make her aware of the abnormal x-ray? Yes, despite the absence of a physician-patient relationship, he should have acted to make her aware of the abnormality that was potentially life threatening.

Case Discussion 4: Sexual Act with Patient

An emergency department nursing assistant allegedly engaged in digital and oral sex with a patient without resistance. The patient stated while the assistant was alone in the room with her, she made sexual comments to get him to release her from restraints. She had been brought in by police for a manic-depressive disorder and was yelling, kicking, and swearing and had to be restrained. The patient told a social worker about the sexual incident 3 days later.

Legal issue: Was the medical center liable for the actions of the nursing assistant under the theory of *respondeat superior*?

Disposition: The jury at the trial court level awarded the plaintiff $750,000 for past damages and $500,000 for future damages. The verdict was reduced to present-day value and a judgment was rendered for $1,147,247.42. The court of appeals reversed and remanded the case for entry of a judgment of dismissal holding that the trial court erred in denying directed verdict and motion for summary judgment because the plaintiff failed to present a material question of fact regarding the defendant's liability under the legal doctrine of *respondeat superior*. The Supreme Court of Michigan held that the court of appeals correctly reversed the trial court judgment. The plaintiff did not prove the defendant was liable under the doctrine of *respondeat superior*. The nursing assistant was not acting within the scope of his employment when he engaged in sexual acts with the plaintiff.[2]

---

[1]*Stanley v. McCarver*, No. CV-03-0099-PR (D. Ariz. Filed June 29, 2004).
[2]*Zsigo v. Hurley Med. Ctr.*, 716 N.W.2d 220 (Mich. 2006).

Case Discussion 5: Radioiodine Therapy for Pregnant Patient

In *Bentley v. Riverside Community Hospital*[1] the court held that the plaintiffs failed to meet their burden of presenting sufficient evidence to prove that the hospital personnel had a duty to ask the patient whether she was pregnant immediately before the radiologist administered radioiodine therapy to treat symptoms of Graves disease, or hyperthyroidism. The court concluded that it was the physician's duty to obtain informed consent for the radioiodine therapy and it was not delegable.

Case Discussion 6: Treatment of Suicidal Patient

A patient was admitted to the defendant hospital's behavioral science unit 1 day after slitting his wrist in an attempted suicide. The patient continued having suicidal thoughts while in the defendant hospital. Four days after admission, the patient used a plastic garbage can liner that was in the room and suffocated himself. The hospital's employees performed as many as 12 bed checks while the patient lay dead in his bed. The patient's death was only discovered when the hospital's staff attempted to awaken him the following morning. The Pennsylvania jury found that the hospital and the defendant physician, who treated the patient a decade earlier for depression, were grossly negligent in treating the decedent. The plaintiff received $800,000 in compensatory damages from both defendants and $800,000 in punitive damages against the hospital.[2] (Punitive damages are designed to punish the healthcare provider for conduct that is considered to be grossly negligent. Insurance policies usually do not provide coverage for punitive damages, so these awards are paid out of the pocket of the defendant.)

Case Discussion 7: Dental Surgery Follow-Up

A 60-year-old Georgia truck driver had a wisdom tooth extracted by the defendant dentist. Several weeks later, another dentist diagnosed osteomyelitis (bone infection) and pathological fracture (fracture from a weakened bone) of the patient's lower jaw secondary to a postoperative infection. Surgery had to be performed to remove decayed tissue and bone and to wire the jaw. Other treatment required included intravenous antibiotics, hyperbaric oxygen treatments, and bone grafting to the jaw.

The plaintiff claimed that the extraction was unnecessary and that the defendant failed to give him appropriate postextraction instructions and to diagnose the infection during postoperative visits. The defendant contended that the extraction was necessary, that the plaintiff did not take the antibiotics as instructed, and that he did not keep all follow-up appointments. The verdict was for the defense.[3] In this case, the specific recording of missed appointments by the office staff of the dentist was a key factor in defending the dentist.

---

[1]*Bentley v. Riverside Comm. Hosp.,* No. E037566 (Cal. App. Dist. 4 July 31, 2006).
[2]Laska L, editor: Pennsylvania man used garbage can bag to commit suicide, *Medical Malpractice Verdicts, Settlements and Experts,* 43, January 1996.
[3]Laska L, editor: Georgia man develops severe infection after extraction of wisdom tooth, *Medical Malpractice Verdicts, Settlements and Experts,* 8, February 1996.

Case Discussion 8: Dental Diagnosis and Treatment

A woman in her early thirties alleged that her dentist was negligent in failing to diagnose and treat periodontal disease and in failing to perform pocket depth probing or take x-rays. The defendant contended that the plaintiff declined x-rays because of the cost and that she did refer the plaintiff to a periodontist. The dentist added to her defense by maintaining that the plaintiff was contributorily negligent in missing dental appointments and that any delay in diagnosis did not affect outcome. The jury returned a defense verdict.[1]

Case Discussion 9: Alleged Injury during Treadmill Test

A 60-year-old retired woman underwent a stress echocardiogram, which included a treadmill test. A week after the treadmill test, which was done in the cardiologist's office, the woman's husband called the physician to report that she had seriously injured her back when she fell off the treadmill during the test. Neither the cardiologist nor the two technicians present in the room during the test remembered a fall or any other unusual incident occurring at the time. The plaintiff claimed that the technician had negligently instructed her to get off the treadmill while the belt was moving backward, causing her to fall and to suffer a herniated disk. The defendants contended that the plaintiff injured her back sometime after the test and denied that the incident reported by the plaintiff ever happened. The verdict was for the defense.[2]

The defense of the cardiologist and the technicians was based on the premise that the lack of documentation of the alleged fall indicated that it did not occur. An injury of this nature would have been recorded in the cardiologist's office notes. Additional statements by the technicians would have also been appropriate.

Case Discussion 10: Torn Rotator Cuff

A man in his late sixties had a stroke affecting his left side. He claimed that the day after his admission, a radiology technician arrived in his room to transport the man to the radiology department for a test. The plaintiff claimed that the technician reached over and grabbed his flaccid left arm to get him onto the stretcher, resulting in a torn rotator cuff of the left shoulder. The plaintiff's family members, who were in the room at the time, claimed that they complained to the attending nurse, head nurse, and head physician—none of whom had any recollection of the complaint. There was no documentation of a complaint. The defendant denied the incident happened. The defendant also disputed that the event occurred because the rotator cuff tear was not diagnosed until 1 year later.[3] The jury returned a defense verdict.

---

[1]Laska L, editor: Failure to diagnose periodontal disease, *Medical Malpractice Verdicts, Settlements and Experts,* 7, April 1999.
[2]Laska L, editor: California woman claims she fell off treadmill during stress test and injured back, *Medical Malpractice Verdicts, Settlements and Experts,* 6, February 1996.
[3]Laska L, editor: Technician blamed for torn rotator cuff while loading patient on stretcher, *Medical Malpractice Verdicts, Settlements and Experts,* 22, April 1999.

Case Discussion 11: Misplaced MRI

A Texas jury awarded $67.5 million to a child who lost her left leg after her magnetic resonance imaging (MRI) result was misplaced for more than 1 day. After a burro attacked her, the child underwent surgery to remove part of her intestine. A blood clot had formed on her aorta, cutting off circulation to her leg. The plaintiffs argued that if the results of the MRI test had not been lost for more than a day, the clot could have been detected and the leg saved.[1]

The accurate filing of reports is an essential responsibility of all staff members who handle medical records. Paying attention to detail, ensuring that the results are not placed on the wrong person's chart, and properly handling the report are important in managing medical records.

Case Discussion 12: Misplaced Mammogram Report

In a Pennsylvania case, a 48-year-old woman underwent a mammogram in her gynecologist's office under the direction of Spectrascan employees. A Spectrascan employee misdirected the mammogram report to a pile for routine screening tests rather than the pile for diagnostic tests. The plaintiff claimed that her breast cancer was not diagnosed between February 1995 and October 1995, allowing the cancer to spread to her bones, lungs, and brain. She was not expected to survive. A $33.1 million verdict was reached, with the gynecologist and his practice found 17% at fault and Spectrascan found 83% at fault. The verdict included about $1.1 million in past and future medical expenses and lost wages and $27 million to the plaintiff for pain and suffering. Her husband was awarded $5 million for loss of consortium.[2]

Case Discussion 13: Recordkeeping at Nursing Home

A Florida woman died in a nursing home after having been a patient for 5 years. She was 94 years old at the time of admission. During her stay, she was totally dependent on skilled nursing and catheter care, but the level of care was apparently very poor. Recordkeeping was severely deficient—sometimes with gaps of weeks between the required daily nursing notes. Existing notes were often internally conflicting or in conflict with other pieces of the decedent's chart that other caretakers had recorded on the same day. The woman suffered a broken ankle, broken hip, torn rotator cuff, numerous stage IV bedsores (the most serious type), and severe contractures while in the home. She died of congestive heart failure, with sepsis (blood infection) listed as a secondary cause of death. Two days before trial, the parties settled for $800,000.[3] Frequency of charting was an issue in this case.

[1]Laska L, editor: Lost MRI blamed for failure to detect blood clot, resulting in child's loss of left leg and damage to nerves in right leg, *Medical Malpractice Verdicts, Settlements and Experts,* 18, August 1999.
[2]Laska L, editor: Mammogram report put in wrong pile, *Medical Malpractice Verdicts, Settlements and Experts,* 21, August 1999.
[3]Laska L, editor: Elderly woman dies in nursing home, *Medical Malpractice Verdicts, Settlements and Experts,* 26-27, January 1996.

Case Discussion 14: Testing Errors

Blood tests were ordered for a patient suffering symptoms of weakness in her lower extremities. The tests were to determine if she had multiple sclerosis or a vitamin B_{12} deficiency. The laboratory incorrectly reported a normal range for vitamin B_{12} as a result of an error in methodology. Vitamin B_{12} tests were ordered again because the patient's symptoms worsened, but the tests were never performed. The patient became permanently paralyzed.

The error in testing methodology resulted in a $10 million verdict for the patient, and the laboratory and the hospital were both held to be 50% responsible for the plaintiff's resulting paralysis and damages.[1]

---

[3]*National Health Laboratories v. Pari*, 596 A.2d 555 (D.C. 1991).

Case Studies

Case Study 1: EMT Liability for Death

Are EMTs who have disconnected oxygen liable for the death of a terminally ill patient?

FACTS: The deceased patient was a nursing home resident for 8 years who had multiple chronic conditions, including diabetic ketoacidosis, rheumatoid arthritis with Felty's syndrome, hypothyroidism, diverticulitis, multiple endocrine neoplasia syndrome no. 1, left nephrectomy with left staghorn calculus removal, hiatal hernia with esophageal reflux, and multiple drug allergies. She was transferred to a hospital for acute care of severe, intractable nausea as well as vomiting and possible starvation. At the request of her family, a do-not-resuscitate (DNR) order had been on the patient's chart for 5 years. She was unable to take anything by mouth, but the family declined insertion of a feeding tube. While in the hospital, the patient suffered a significant drop in blood pressure that was initially treated with IV dopamine. The family requested that the medication be discontinued after 1 day. Over the following week, the patient's condition declined rapidly; she was nonresponsive and had difficulty breathing. She was receiving oxygen by nasal cannula but no other treatment. Because her condition was terminal, the decision was made to transfer her back to the nursing home, with the family's consent. The defendant ambulance service was called by the hospital to transfer the patient back to the nursing home. While moving the patient from her bed to the ambulance, the emergency medical technicians discontinued the oxygen. It is disputed whether the oxygen was administered during the 7-minute ride to the nursing home. Upon arrival and transfer of the patient to the nursing home, she was no longer breathing. The patient's children filed a malpractice case against the ambulance company and the EMTs.[1]

Case Study 1 Questions

1. Is there any factual basis for asserting a malpractice claim?
2. What impact does the DNR order have upon the analysis?
3. Do the patient's numerous terminal conditions affect the family's right to recover damages? If so, how?

---

[1]*Alphonse v. Acadian Ambulance Services, Inc.*, 844 So.2d 294 (La. 2003).

Case Study 2: Informed Consent

Does a student or preceptor have a duty to obtain informed consent?

FACTS: A few weeks before the plaintiff was to have a vaginal hysterectomy, she told her gynecologist that she preferred privacy during her surgery. To this end, she crossed out two portions of the physician's consent form before she signed it: she crossed out "I consent to the presence of healthcare learners" and "I consent to the photography o[r] videotaping of the surgical, diagnostic, and/or medical procedure to be performed providing my name and identity is not revealed." On the morning that her surgery was to be performed, the plaintiff received assurance from the attending anesthesiologist that she would personally be handling her anesthesia. The anesthesiologist's consent form, which the plaintiff signed, read in part: "I understand that my anesthesia care will be given to me by the undersigned or a physician privileged to practice anesthesia." After the plaintiff was anesthetized, a hospital employee, acting as a preceptor, entered the operating room with a student in an emergency medical technician (EMT) certification program. The anesthesiologist granted permission for the EMT student to intubate the plaintiff. During the unsuccessful intubation, the plaintiff's esophagus was torn.[1]

Case Study 2 Questions

1. Who had the duty to obtain and conform to the informed consent given by the plaintiff?
2. Did the student have a duty to review the patient consent form before the attempted intubation?
3. Did the preceptor have a duty to review the signed consent form?
4. Was the attempted intubation considered battery?

Case Study 3: Intentional Tort

Is an intentional tort malpractice?

FACTS: In June 2004, the plaintiff sought treatment at the defendant's hospital. After conducting both physical and psychological examinations, the plaintiff's physicians determined that he was at risk of committing suicide and should be restrained. Because the plaintiff refused to cooperate with nurses or security guards, hospital employees forcibly strapped him to a gurney. On June 28, 2006, the plaintiff filed suit alleging that the defendant, through its agents, servants, or employees, committed false imprisonment, assault, and battery. The court dismissed the case because the plaintiff had not complied with the procedural requirement of medical malpractice law. On appeal, the plaintiff asserts that the trial court erred in determining that his complaint alleged a cause of action for medical malpractice.[2]

Case Study 3 Questions

1. Was the trial correct in determining that intentional torts in a hospital setting are malpractice?
2. What two critical factors determine whether a claim is medical malpractice?

[1]*Mullins v. Parkview Hospital, Inc.*, 830 N.E.2d 45 (Ind. Ct. App. 2005).
[2]*Brown v. Henry Ford Health Systems*, Docket No. 273441 (Mich. May 3, 2007).

Case Study 4: Intentional Tort

Who is liable for the intentional torts of hospital staff?

FACTS: A female patient was admitted to a hospital ICU in a diminished mental and physical condition. She claimed that the medications she was given keep her in an impaired mental state. She alleged that while in the ICU in this diminished capacity, she was sexually assaulted by a male registered nurse.[*] The patient sued the hospital for assault, battery, and intentional infliction of emotional distress.[1] Although the patient could have named the assailant in this case, the plaintiff did not sue him. Is the hospital liable as the employer?

Case Study 4 Questions

1. What is the difference between assault and battery?
2. Under what theory could a hospital be liable for the actions of its employees?
3. What does "in the scope of employment" mean?
4. Are there exceptions to the general rule?
5. What implication does the result in this case have with respect to employees maintaining their own malpractice insurance?

Case Study 5: Laboratory Results

Does a laboratory have an affirmative duty to disclose positive HIV test results?

FACTS: The plaintiffs were a husband and wife who tested positive for HIV in a life insurance application physical. The independent laboratory reported the HIV status to the insurance company, which sent a notice of rejection to the couple. The insurance company also advised that it would disclose the reason for their rejection to their physician if they so wished. The plaintiffs took no action. Two years later, the wife was diagnosed with AIDS, and on inquiry, she and her husband learned that insurance company records showed the positive HIV result from 2 years earlier. The plaintiffs sued, alleging that the defendants were negligent in failing to tell them they were HIV positive. When the lab reported the plaintiffs' HIV status to the insurer, the results were also reported to the Kansas Department of Health, as required by Kansas law. In its letter denying coverage, the insurance company advised each plaintiff that the applications were denied on the basis of blood results and offered to send the results to the couple's physician upon written authorization, stating: "With your approval, we would be willing to send the results of the blood profile to your physician so that you can discuss the findings with them. Please write the name and address of the physician you want the blood report sent to at the bottom of this letter and return it to me in the enclosed envelope." The plaintiffs made no inquiry until the wife developed AIDS symptoms in June 2001, at which point they contacted the insurance company and asked it to release the blood test results to their physicians. The company duly complied with the request.[2]

---

[*]The assailant could have been a lab or respiratory technician, or other ancillary healthcare personnel.
[1]*Salinas v. Genesys Health System*, 688 N.W.2d 112 (Mich. App. 2004). For another court's opinion on a similar issue, see *N.X., Plaintiff vs. Cabrini Medical Center*, 719 N.Y.S.2d 60 (N.Y. Slip Op. 00432 2001).
[2]*Pehle v. Farm Bureau*, 397 F.3d 897 (10th Cir. 2005).

Case Study 5 Questions

1. Does an independent laboratory hired by an insurance company have a duty to disclose the results of blood tests to policy applicants?
2. What is the difference between the duties of the laboratory and those of the insurance company, if any, and why?
3. Does it make a difference who hired the person responsible for the blood draw? Why or why not?

Case Study 6: Legal Obligations of an Educational Facility

What is the legal obligation of an educational facility to its students?

FACTS: In September 1994, a student entered into a contract for educational services with Yale University to pursue a degree in its pediatric nurse practitioner program (PNPP). Under the terms of the contract, the student was required to complete 18 courses and a research praxis. In April 1996, the student was required to submit her proposed topic for her research praxis to her faculty advisers. The student claimed that from September 1996 through January 1997, she requested that an adviser assist her in the following manner: (a) to discuss the research the plaintiff had already completed in order to narrow the scope of the ongoing research and enable the plaintiff to set successful parameters for her research; (2) to review the sources already used and to suggest appropriate sources for research material going forward; (3) to review and critique drafts for content, clarity, scope, and further research that was to be recommended; and (4) to provide necessary advisory services to the plaintiff. After the unsuccessful completion of the research project, the student filed suit against the university, alleging that it denied her request for educational services when her advisers left the school in January and April 1996, respectively, without leaving any notes, memoranda, written analyses, or any other forms of communication that would assist the plaintiff and/or her successive advisors in completing the research praxis. The student also claimed that there were periods of time, totaling several months, in which she had to complete the research praxis without assistance from an adviser and that such interruptions in supervision and advisorship hindered her performance and prevented her from successfully completing her research praxis. In essence, the student alleged that (a) the defendants breached their performance obligations under the educational agreement; (b) she suffered damages in that she has incurred significant debt because she has not been able to obtain employment in her specialized area without completion of the degree program; and (c) the defendants intentionally inflicted emotional distress because they knew or should have known that their conduct would create an unreasonable risk of causing emotional distress and that such emotional distress would reasonably result in illness or bodily harm to the plaintiff.[1]

Case Study 6 Questions

1. Did the university breach its performance obligations under the terms of the educational agreement with the student?
2. What are the limits of a university's obligations to its students regarding required courses?

---

[1]*Superior Court of Connecticut, Judicial District of Hartford,* Super. LEXIS 1583 (unreported) (Conn. 2003).

Case Study 7: Medical Product Liability

What are the limits on medical product liability cases under federal law?

FACTS: On May 10, 1996, the plaintiff underwent a percutaneous transluminal coronary angioplasty, intended to dilate his right coronary artery, which had been found to be "diffusely diseased" and "heavily calcified." The physician used an Evergreen balloon catheter, which is specifically contraindicated for patients who have "diffuse or calcified stenoses." During the procedure, the physician first attempted to remove the calcium deposits in the plaintiff's artery with a Rotoblator device, and then unsuccessfully inserted several different balloon catheters. The physician ultimately inserted the Evergreen balloon catheter into the patient's artery and inflated the device several times, up to a pressure of 10 atmospheres. The device label for the Evergreen balloon catheter specifies that it should not be inflated beyond the "rated burst pressure" of 8 atmospheres. On the final inflation, the balloon catheter burst, and the plaintiff began to rapidly deteriorate. He developed a complete heart block, lost consciousness, was intubated and placed on advanced life support, and was rushed to the operating room for emergency coronary bypass surgery. The plaintiff survived, but according to his complaint suffered "severe and permanent personal injuries and disabilities." The patient filed suit against the manufacturer, alleging strict liability; breach of implied warranty; and negligent design, testing, inspection, distribution, labeling, marketing, sale, and manufacture.[1] The Evergreen balloon catheter entered the market pursuant to the Food and Drug Administration's (FDA) premarket approval process in the mid-1990s. The warning and contraindications for use of the catheter were clearly noted on the product information label.

Case Study 7 Questions

1. What is the FDA premarket approval process?
2. How does the FDA's premarket approval process affect lawsuits that allege injuries caused by defective medical devices?
3. What does a plaintiff have to prove to win a case against the manufacturer of a premarket-approved medical device?

Case Study 8: Mobile Screening Unit Duties

Does the healthcare provider have a duty to inform a screened employee of abnormal test results?

FACTS: In December 1994, Mobile Medical entered into a contract with the city of Yonkers to provide physical examinations to firefighters employed by the Yonkers fire department and, on the basis of those examinations, to determine whether the firefighters were fit for duty. The physical examinations consisted of an electrocardiogram (ECG), a pulmonary function test, and a fitness test, each performed by qualified medical technicians under physician supervision. Mobile Medical personnel performed a physical examination of the plaintiff to evaluate his ability to continue working with the fire department. Following the administration of the ECG, the plaintiff asked the physician about the results of his test and received the following response: "Everything looks fine. We only found one irregular heartbeat." The plaintiff did not seek any subsequent medical treatment or additional testing. The plaintiff subsequently suffered a heart attack at his home.[2]

---

[1]*Riegel v. Medtronic, Inc.,* 451 F.3d 104 (2nd Cir., 2006); cert. granted, *Riegel v. Medtronic, Inc.,* 127 S. Ct. 3000.
[2]*Joseph Dugan et al. v. Mobile Medical Testing Services, Inc., et al.,* 830 A.2d 752 (Conn. 2003).

Case Study 8 Questions

1. Do a physician and staff hired by an employer to do medical screenings have a physician-patient relationship with the employee?
2. Do the medical screeners have a duty to notify the employee directly of abnormal results?
3. Does the physician's statement to the plaintiff that "he had one irregular heartbeat, but that everything else looked fine" create a duty to inform the plaintiff of an abnormal ECG?

Case Study 9: Ordinary Negligence vs. Malpractice

Is it ordinary negligence or malpractice?

FACTS: When Hurricane Katrina hit New Orleans, Louisiana, in 2005, many hospitalized patients died as a result of flooding, electrical failure, and failure to evacuate patients from hospitals. When the Mayor of New Orleans issued an evacuation order 20 hours before the storm hit, he did not include hospitals and their patients. A day later, the city suffered a power outage and severe flooding; the emergency generators in the hospitals did not respond because they were either in the basement or at ground level and were under water. Ventilator patients were among the first patients to die. The families of deceased patients filed suit in court against the hospital for their family members' deaths. The hospital asked to have the case dismissed because it had not been presented first to the malpractice review panel as required under Louisiana law in malpractice cases involving healthcare. The trial court refused to dismiss the case, saying it was not a medical malpractice case.[1] The appellate court reversed[2] the decision and said the allegations of the failure of timely evacuation and failure to have an emergency plan for the safety of its patients were malpractice, because some measure of medical judgment was required in determining who should be evacuated and when. The appellate court dismissed those claims. The Louisiana Supreme Court agreed to decide the question. The issue before the Louisiana Supreme Court was whether the failure to evacuate or to be prepared for the level of disaster that occurred was malpractice or ordinary negligence.[3]

Case Study 9 Questions

1. Explain the difference between ordinary negligence and professional malpractice.
2. Did the hospital's failure to evacuate or prevent harm in advance to its patients from the consequences of a hurricane involve ordinary care or professional judgment?
3. Does it make a difference that the hospital was located in a hurricane-prone area that lies below sea level?

---

[1]*Stephen B. LaCoste, et al., v. Pendleton Methodist Hospital, L.L.C.,* 2006 WL 4544796 (La. Civil D. Ct. August 30, 2006).
[2]*LaCoste v. Pendleton Methodist Hospital, L.L.C.,* 947 So.2d 150 (La. App. December 6, 2006).
[3]*LaCoste v. Pendleton,* 2007 WL 2482676 (La. September 5, 2007).

Case Study 10: Privacy

Is disclosure of a patient's confession to a crime a violation of the right to privacy?

FACTS: On May 11, 1998, a masked gunman, the defendant, robbed a bank. The following day, he contacted a clinic seeking an emergency appointment with a psychiatric nurse practitioner who had been involved with his therapy for 1 or 2 years. During the appointment, the gunman told his psychiatric nurse practitioner, "I done something very stupid," and that he did not want to "go to jail." He gave an envelope to the psychiatric nurse practitioner and told her to give it to his daughter. He then said that he had overdosed on his medications. The psychiatric nurse practitioner was concerned that the defendant was suicidal, and she wanted to telephone for an ambulance. The man protested that he did not want the police contacted because he had robbed a bank and had been burned when "the money exploded." He lifted his shirt to show her the burn marks on his stomach. He also had a gun that he voluntarily turned over to the psychiatric nurse practitioner, again stating he did not want to go to jail. He asked the psychiatric nurse practitioner not to tell anyone. Although the psychiatric nurse practitioner had not contacted the police, the ambulance company had notified the police that an ambulance was en route to the clinic to attend to a suspected drug overdose. An officer was dispatched to assist the ambulance crew if necessary and remained behind at the clinic to speak to the psychiatric nurse practitioner and the gunman's former girlfriend, who had arrived. The girlfriend told the police that her boyfriend said he had robbed a bank, and the psychiatric nurse practitioner subsequently confirmed the statement. After his arrest and arraignment, the man claimed that his confession should be suppressed, because it was made to his psychiatric nurse practitioner, who had violated her obligation to keep the information confidential.[1] The applicable law says, "[I]n any court proceeding and in any proceeding preliminary thereto and in legislative and administrative proceedings, a patient shall have the privilege of refusing to disclose, and of preventing a witness from disclosing, any communication, wherever made, between said patient and a psychotherapist relative to the diagnosis or treatment of the patient's mental or emotional condition."

Case Study 10 Questions

1. Does the code of professional ethics affect whether the psychiatric nurse practitioner can ethically testify to the confession at trial?
2. Does the defendant have a valid breach of privacy claim against the psychiatric nurse practitioner for turning the gun over to the police?
3. Are there exceptions to confidentiality requirements that might apply in this case to permit the disclosures?

Case Study 11: *Res Ipsa Loquitur*

Is the doctrine of *res ipsa loquitur* applicable to establish negligence?

FACTS: The patient had been under the care of his family practice physician for 25 years. For 19 of those years, he was quadriplegic as a result of a car accident. He had no use of his lower limbs or his trunk, no use of his right upper limb, and only a very slight range of motion in his left upper extremity. In November 1996, the patient had

---

[1]*Commonwealth of Massachusetts v. Brandein*, 760 N.E.2d 724 (Mass. 2002).

a small lesion removed from his head by his physician. The procedure was done in an examination room at the physician's office, with the assistance of the office nurse. Before the procedure, the patient was transferred from his wheelchair to the examining table by his wife, who then left the room. The examining table had no side rails or restraints. There was a dispute about the positioning of the plaintiff on the examination table, but when the patient later fell, there was no question that he had fallen. The patient later died. While still alive, before trial, the patient testified in a deposition that the nurse and physician positioned him on the examination table on his right side with a pillow behind his back, under his head, and between his knees. No one was present in the room at the time of the fall. The patient did not know exactly how or why he fell, but he testified that after being left lying on his right side, he felt his body roll to the right and fall to the floor. The nurse and physician claim they left the patient lying on his back in the middle of the examination table. The plaintiff asked the judge to instruct the jury that they could infer, from the circumstances of the case, that the defendants had been negligent. This instruction is the doctrine of *res ipsa loquitur*. This phrase is Latin for "the thing speaks for itself." In most states, this doctrine only applies when the defendant is the sole person in control of the "instrumentality" that caused the harm. It is most often applied in malpractice cases involving surgical errors, because the plaintiff is unconscious and has no way of knowing what actually happened, and the operating staff are totally in control of the patient's well-being and the environment. *Res ipsa loquitur* allows a jury to find the defendant(s) responsible for the harm if all other possible causes have been excluded, even though plaintiffs have no direct evidence of the defendant's negligence. The trial court judge did not allow the jury to infer negligence, explaining that the plaintiff's wife had failed to establish either that the fall from the examination table was "of the kind that usually does not occur in the absence of negligence" or that other causes, such as the patient's own conduct, were eliminated by the evidence. On appeal, the court ruled that a quadriplegic could not normally fall from an examination table absent negligence, and that, in this case, other causes for the fall were eliminated. Thus, the appeals court concluded that the jury should have been allowed to infer negligence and reversed the verdict. The Supreme Court of Pennsylvania agreed to hear the case to determine whether the doctrine of *res ipsa loquitur* applies in this case.[1]

Case Study 11 Questions

1. Should the judge have given the *res ipsa loquitur* instruction to the jury in this case?
2. Is there any evidence of how the fall occurred? Could it have occurred in the absence of negligence?
3. Can all causes of the fall other than the defendant's negligence be ruled out with no evidence presented to establish what actually happened?

Case Study 12: Respiratory Therapy/Radiology

Who committed malpractice?

FACTS: The plaintiff was seriously injured in a single-vehicle accident in which he sustained a mild to moderate concussion and multiple facial fractures. Upon arriving at the trauma center at the hospital nearly 4 hours after the accident, the plaintiff had a blood alcohol level of 0.13%, which extrapolated to approximately 0.20% at

---

[1]*Quinby v. Plumsteadville Family Practice, Inc.*, 907 A.2d 1061 (Pa. 2006).

the time of the accident. The plaintiff was connected to a ventilator to assist his breathing and remained on a ventilator while at the hospital. Over the next 2 days, the plaintiff remained in stable condition but suffered from "severe agitation." The plaintiff was given unusually large doses of Valium, fentanyl, and other drugs to keep him sedated from his presumed alcohol withdrawal. CT scans were ordered in preparation for reconstructive surgery to treat the plaintiff's facial fractures. A registered nurse, a respiratory therapist, and a nurse's aide prepared to transport the plaintiff to radiology and connected the plaintiff to a portable cardiac monitor and to a portable ventilator. The ventilator was attached to one of three portable oxygen tanks that accompanied plaintiff to the CT suite. One of the tanks was full, and the remaining tanks were half full. The respiratory therapist did not record the portable ventilator's settings and alarm parameters before leaving the neurological intensive care unit. The nurse did not verify the alarms or the parameters on the plaintiff's portable cardiac monitor or make any entry in his medical record of either the alarm parameters or the patient's vital signs. Upon arriving at the CT suite, the nurse administered a paralytic drug to the plaintiff in preparation for the CT scans. As a result, the plaintiff was unable to move or breathe on his own and became completely dependent on the portable ventilator. The nurse never informed the other healthcare providers that she had administered the drug. From the control room, the nurse and respiratory therapist could see the CT table through a glass window and could observe the plaintiff's face on a television monitor. Neither looked at the cardiac monitor or the ventilator while the plaintiff was in the CT scanner. The nurse testified that she was watching the plaintiff's face and was listening for alarms. Both she and the respiratory therapist testified that no alarms ever sounded. They both testified that the plaintiff's complexion was "pink" and that he was breathing when he exited the scanner. Shortly after the plaintiff was returned to bed, someone noticed that he had turned gray and was not breathing. Although successfully resuscitated, he sustained severe and permanent brain damage.[1]

Case Study 12 Questions

1. What were the breaches of the standard of care?
2. Was the nurse responsible for the actions/inactions of the respiratory therapist?
3. Was the nurse's failure to communicate the administration of a paralytic drug a legal cause of the brain damage; if so, did it change the respiratory therapist's duties to the patient?
4. Did the radiology technician breach a duty to the plaintiff?

Case Study 13: Spoliation

How does the spoliation of evidence affect a lawsuit?

FACTS: The plaintiff began receiving treatment at the hospital in March 1997 for an abscess in his left groin. During a surgical procedure to drain the abscess on March 16, 1997, the surgeon found several areas of necrotic tissue and proceeded to débride the dead material. The plaintiff was prescribed the antibiotics Rocephin and gentamicin to treat the infection. The surgeon sent a sample of the removed tissue to be cultured and tested for "sensitivities" to antibiotics. The hospital performed the requested tests and reported that one source of the infection, group B *Streptococcus,*

[1]*Mercer v. Vanderbilt University, Inc.,* 134 S.W.3d 121 (Tenn. 2004).

was "sensitive" to the antibiotic ciprofloxacin. Following receipt of the lab report, the plaintiff's medication was changed to ciprofloxacin. On March 19, a second débridement was performed and a diagnosis of necrotizing fasciitis, also known as Fournier's gangrene, was made. Additional blood work, chest x-rays, and a glucose tolerance test were ordered and the plaintiff was discharged. He returned to the emergency department 4 days later, seeking treatment for continued drainage and irritation in the groin area. A second physician discontinued the ciprofloxacin and ordered Unasyn in its place. However, because the necrosis had severely progressed before the medication change, continued débridement ultimately resulted in the loss of the plaintiff's entire penis. All the tissue débrided in these procedures was discarded rather than sent to the hospital's laboratory for testing. The plaintiff alleged that if the débrided tissue had been tested microbiologically, the tests might have shown that the group B *Streptococcus* infection was still active, and his medication could have been changed at that time. He contends that the lack of these laboratory tests was equivalent to missing evidence that prevented him from proving an essential element of his case against the hospital. Under Kentucky law, a hospital has a duty to examine "tissues removed at surgery." There is an exception for "[s]pecimens that by their nature or condition do not permit fruitful examination." The court gave the "missing evidence" instruction to the jury.[1]

Case Study 13 Questions

1. What is a missing evidence instruction and how does it affect a case?
2. Was there a duty to preserve this evidence?
3. Who was responsible for the failure to preserve evidence: the hospital, the physicians, or both?

Case Study 14: Statute of Limitations

Does a plaintiff healthcare professional have a greater duty to discover a potential claim for malpractice for purposes of the statute of limitations?

FACTS: On March 9, 1993, the plaintiff suffered from a sore neck while at work as a nurse anesthetist at the hospital. The pain increased throughout the day and, after having difficulty sleeping because of the pain, the plaintiff visited the emergency department at the hospital in the early morning of March 10, 1993. While in the emergency department, the plaintiff was examined by a physician, who suggested that the plaintiff undergo a computerized axial tomography (CAT) scan. After undergoing the CAT scan, the plaintiff subsequently was discharged from the hospital by another emergency department physician. The discharge papers indicated that the CAT scan had revealed a possible brain bulge, cerebral edema, and cervical arthritis. Also, upon being discharged, the plaintiff was prescribed medication that he knew was used to reduce brain swelling. After being discharged from the emergency department, the plaintiff returned to his home. Thereafter, on March 12, 1993, the plaintiff awoke and noticed strange temperature sensations in his hands. Subsequently, the plaintiff realized that he was unable to hold a pen or write, and he experienced other subtle changes in motor control functions. At that time, the plaintiff returned to the emergency department of the hospital, where the defendant physician ordered another CAT scan. The plaintiff was then admitted to the hospital and on March 16, 1993, the plaintiff

---

[1] *Rogers et al., v. T.J. Samson Community Hospital,* 276 F.3d 228 (6th Cir. 2002).

was told by a neurologist, Yolanda Pena, that he had suffered a stroke on March 12. The plaintiff testified that he did not question the care he had received at the hospital until 1995, when he read two magazine articles regarding the treatment of strokes. As a result of reading those articles, the plaintiff, in October 1995, sought legal counsel regarding the treatment he had received at the hospital. The plaintiff also testified that the first time that he read his emergency department record from March 10, 1993, was when he met with his legal counsel. That record revealed that the physician had recorded his diagnosis of the plaintiff as including a "possible [cerebrovascular accident] CVA." The statute of limitations that is applicable to this action provides that a person must bring an action within 2 years from the date that he discovers, or in the exercise of reasonable care should have discovered, that he has suffered actionable harm.[1]

Case Study 14 Questions

1. What is the purpose of the statute of limitations?
2. Do education, knowledge, and/or experience in a healthcare field create an obligation to investigate possible malpractice earlier than for non-healthcare providers?
3. When did the statute of limitations start to run in this case?

---

[1] *Winsted Memorial Hospital et al.,* 817 A.2d 619 (Conn. 2003).

Supplemental Case Scenarios

Case Scenario 1: Student's Unsatisfactory Performance

Allen is a dental hygienist student in his last year of college at a state institution. Allen has met with his adviser several times, who informed him, in writing and orally, that his clinical skills were not "up to par." His adviser stated on one occasion that "if he did not improve, he was in danger of being on probation or being dismissed from the program." Allen knows that he has been having difficulty in the clinical area. He argues that his clinical instructor, Brenda South, does not "like him." Three weeks before the end of the semester, May 30, the department informed Allen that he would not graduate as expected on June 15. The department chair indicated that Allen's "clinical skills were unsatisfactory and his performance was below that of other students in his class." Allen is very upset and challenges the decision.

What are the responsibilities of the chair? What are the responsibilities of the adviser and the clinical instructor? What are Allen's rights? Does he have any? What laws allow Allen to file a lawsuit against the faculty challenging the faculty's evaluation and dismissal decision? What process is due to ensure that fairness prevails?

Case Scenario 2: Signing Consent Forms

Mrs. Richards is an elderly woman who is in the advanced stages of Alzheimer's disease. Her husband has been noticing that lately his wife has had bloody stools. On Tuesday, Mrs. Richards comes to the hospital for a colonoscopy procedure to rule out colon cancer. Susan White is the radiology technician working in the radiology department that day. When Mrs. Richards arrives with her husband, Susan escorts them into a waiting area. Susan notes that the consent form for the procedure has not been signed. Susan hands the form to Mrs. Richards and asks her to sign it. Mr. Richards takes the form out of his wife's hands and says that he has always made the decisions in their family and that he is going to sign the form. He then proceeds to ask Susan to explain the potential risks and side effects of the procedure. She attempts to answer his questions as best she can.

What should Susan do? Can the patient's husband sign the consent form?

Case Scenario 3: Patient Noncompliance

A nurse's aide in a hospital is making rounds to pick up lunch trays. An elderly patient has not eaten her food again. The aide asks if the patient wants her lunch to be reheated.

The patient shakes her head no and says, "Please just tell them I ate everything. I don't want any more food. I just want to die." The aide leaves the room with the tray but is upset. Without food, the patient will starve to death.

If the aide lies to the nurse at the patient's request, is she helping the patient commit suicide? Can a competent adult refuse to eat? Is the patient competent?

Case Scenario 4: Anesthetic for Brain-Damaged Patient

A certified nursing assistant has been employed by a family to take care of a 7-year-old girl severely brain damaged in a near-drowning accident when she was 3 years old. During the 3 months the assistant has been employed, she has had the opportunity to know the young patient well. Although the girl cannot talk, the nursing assistant has learned about the foods her patient likes and dislikes, that the girl sleeps better if she is placed on her right side, that she cries whenever she hears loud noises, and that she likes to listen to music. One day, the nursing assistant accompanies the patient and her mother to a physician's office for minor surgery on the child's hand to remove a small cyst. The physician asks the nursing assistant to stay with the child to help hold her hand in position while the minor surgery is completed. The assistant notices that the physician is not preparing to give the child an anesthetizing injection on her arm, where the surgery is to be done. She asks about this, and the physician states, "She doesn't need anything. She's just a vegetable."

What should the assistant do?

Case Scenario 5: Treatment and Religious Freedom

A medical assistant is employed in an oncologist's office. He greets a patient he knows well, a 62-year-old woman with leukemia. Her blood work shows that her white blood cell (WBC) count is down. The assistant gives this result to the physician, who orders an infusion of fresh frozen plasma (FFP). The assistant reminds the physician that the patient is a Jehovah's Witness, a religious group that refuses all blood products, including FFP, in treatment. The physician becomes angry. "Just tell her it's medicine that I ordered. Don't tell her it's a blood product. It's not red, so she'll never guess. It's the only thing I have that can help her right now." Should the medical assistant lie to the patient at the request of the physician? Either he must obey the physician and lie or refuse to reveal to the patient that the physician has ordered a blood product for her, or he must disobey the physician and inform the patient that her treatment is a blood product. His only other option is to leave the office, which will cost him his job and still not assist the patient. The medical assistant must make a choice.

Are the options being considered respectful or disrespectful of the patient's autonomy? What should the assistant do? Are there potential legal implications?

Case Scenario 6: Patient Privacy

A high school student studying in a health professions course at school spends a day following a nurse in her practice in an obstetrics-gynecology clinic. While at the clinic, a classmate patient is treated and recognized by the student. The patient is pregnant and is upset and unsure about what to do about her pregnancy. The nurse, with the student watching and listening, spends a lot of time counseling the patient. Later, another classmate stops the health professions student and says, "I saw you with Didi in the clinic. What was she in for? Is she pregnant?"

Should the health professions student reveal the patient's diagnosis? What are the potential legal implications?

Case Scenario 7: Administering Incorrect Medication

Marcia Logan, RT (ARRT), was preparing Mr. Samuel for a fluoroscopic x-ray examination of his lower intestine, also called a barium enema study. Soon after Marcia inserted the enema catheter into Mr. Samuel's rectum, he showed signs of distress. When Marcia asked whether he was all right, he did not respond. Marcia called the radiologist, Dr. Garcia, who was in his office two doors down the hall. Dr. Garcia came immediately, took an intravenous catheter, and prepared to start an IV line for medication administration. He shouted to Marcia to get a bag of normal saline solution for intravenous infusion.

Marcia opened a drawer in the emergency cart and looked for the normal saline solution but did not see any. She did, however, find several bags of a glucose solution that also contained medication. She handed one of these to Dr. Garcia and said, "This is D5W with lidocaine (a heart medication). Is that okay?" Dr. Garcia did not answer. He proceeded to hang the solution bag on an IV pole and connect it to the IV catheter in Mr. Samuel's arm. Within a few seconds, Mr. Samuel became unconscious and suffered a seizure.

Although Mr. Samuel eventually recovered, he sustained brain damage and was not able to return to a normal life. Mr. Samuel sued the hospital, Dr. Garcia, and Marcia Logan.

Who was at fault? Could Marcia have prevented Mr. Samuel's injury? What should she have done? Who breached a standard of care? What are the legal and professional implications?

Case Scenario 8: Employee Privacy

Ester Levin is a health information administrator at North Island Medical Center. David Farmer, the hospital's Vice President of Human Resources, approaches her and requests that Ms. Levin provide him with a printout of certain healthcare records pertaining to Dr. Robert Lewis. Dr. Lewis is employed as a surgical resident at the medical center and was recently hospitalized there. Rumor has it that Dr. Lewis is homosexual and may have tested positive for HIV while hospitalized.

Ms. Levin knows from her training in health information management that information about patients who are HIV positive or diagnosed with acquired immunodeficiency syndrome (AIDS) must be carefully protected. Ms. Levin does not think it appropriate to provide the requested information to Mr. Farmer. Although Mr. Farmer is responsible for hospital personnel, he has never before personally requested hospital records from the patient records department. Ms. Levin asks Mr. Farmer if he has a signed consent form from Dr. Lewis. Mr. Farmer states he does not need one since he is the director of human resources and Dr. Lewis is an employee. Ms. Levin is afraid that if she refuses to provide the requested information she could be disciplined or even lose her job.

What should she do?

Case Scenario 9: Equipment Malfunction

In an effort to alleviate a stricture, a patient had a Foley catheter inserted during surgery. Several days later, healthcare providers discovered a tiny hole in the balloon of the catheter that allowed urine to leak through to the suture line and into the tissue. This situation caused the patient to undergo two additional surgeries.

It is discovered that the negligence was related to a malfunctioning piece of equipment. Janet is puzzled because she reported that piece of faulty equipment to her supervisor.

Who is negligent? Why? What can Janet do? What should Janet have done? How could she have prevented the injury to the patient? What documentation does Janet need to protect herself?

Case Scenario 10: Failure to Monitor Patient

A patient is admitted to Columbus Hospital by his attending physician for complaints of stomach pains. The treating physician knows that the patient has a history of alcohol abuse. The physician orders that the patient be administered the medication Librium on an as-needed basis for any signs of anxiety, which is the first sign of alcohol withdrawal. If alcohol withdrawal is not controlled, the patient can become delusional and cause harm to himself or others. The attending physician has the last actual contact with the patient at 5 PM, at which time he leaves the patient in the hands of the nursing staff.

Although the patient initially does fairly well and is without complaint, his condition deteriorates over time. The night shift staff notices that the patient is experiencing increasing anxiety. The nursing staff does not administer Librium as ordered or call the physician to notify him of the patient's change in condition. The nurses and nurses' aides fail to closely monitor the patient.

The patient's anxiety continues. The patient clearly exhibits unusual or abnormal behavior. The patient verbally expresses anger at himself and others. He advises that he wishes to leave the hospital to buy alcohol. He refuses to comply with nursing instructions. He threatens the other patient in his room with an intravenous pole. The patient's behavior becomes so outrageous that a nurse's aide is placed outside the patient's room to keep a watchful eye on him. The patient's problem continues to escalate and ends when the patient jumps out of the window of his hospital room.

The patient falls several floors and lands on a roof extension below. Emergency services are provided. His life is saved, but he becomes a paraplegic. Before this incident, although he had an active drinking problem, he was a healthy, robust man without physical limitations or mental disability.

Who is negligent? What are the negligent acts?

Case Scenario 11: Discussing Treatment Options

A medical assistant is in the room when the physician discusses with the patient the available treatment and the material risks of having the medical procedure recommended for the treatment of cancer. He notices that the physician fails to discuss the treatment that other physicians have used. When the physician leaves, the patient says that she will just take her chances and not have any treatment.

What should the medical assistant do? Ethically, does he have an obligation to be a patient advocate? What is the ethical dilemma if he discusses other treatment options with the patient?

Case Scenario 12: Advance Directives

A patient is hurried to the operating room for emergency surgery. A coworker says she does not understand why they are trying to save him because he has an advance directive.

What does this coworker need to know about emergency situations and advance directives? Under what circumstances are living wills "null and void" and not followed or enforced by the healthcare providers?

Case Scenario 13: Life-Prolonging Treatment

A patient is dying at home and changes his mind and wants "everything done" including life-prolonging treatment. The healthcare worker hears him but does not convey the message to the family or physician.

What are the ethical implications? What are the potential legal problems that can arise?

Case Scenario 14: Scope of Practice

Louisa Martin is a medical assistant in Portland, Oregon. She has been summoned to a hearing to show cause why she should not be charged with "practicing radiologic technology without a license." When the radiation control officer made an unannounced visit to Dr. Whitfield's medical office, Louisa was in the x-ray room with a patient. The patient was lying on the x-ray table and Louisa was manipulating the dials on the x-ray control panel.

Louisa testifies that she did not practice radiologic technology. "I never pushed the button," she said. "I would prepare the patient and the room for the examination, and then Dr. Whitfield would come by the room and make the exposure."

Louisa is guilty of practicing radiologic technology illegally because Oregon Administrative Rules state: "The 'Practice of Radiologic Technology' shall be defined as but not limited to the use of ionizing radiation upon a human being for diagnostic or therapeutic purposes including the physical positioning of the patient, the determination of exposure parameters, and the handling of the ionizing radiation equipment."

What are the legal and ethical implications?

Case Scenario 15: X-Ray and Diagnosis

Ben is a radiographer and is working the late shift. He is called to the emergency department to take x-rays of an injured wrist. Ben sees what appears to be a fracture through the distal end of the radius, but when he shows the images to Dr. Harcourt, the ED physician, she says, "Just as I thought—perfectly normal." The radiologist is out for the evening and will not see the films until morning. According to ASRT Code of Ethics, Ben is prohibited from making a diagnosis.

What should Ben do?

Case Scenario 16: Distributing Medication

The medication distribution machine requires each healthcare worker's specific identification number to obtain drugs and requires the recording of numbers of those who witness wastage. Julia is new to the unit and notices a list with everyone's identification numbers taped to the back of the machine.

What are the legal implications? What potential problems can arise from this situation?

Case Scenario 17: Alarms and Patient Safety

Rosa, a nursing assistant, enters a patient's room and finds that the alarm is turned off. She mentions it to the nurse in charge, and the nurse tells Rosa to leave it off because it is sounding too often and is "irritating."

What should Rosa do? What are the potential legal and ethical problems? Is this malpractice? Is this providing proper care? Are there disciplinary actions that could result because of a patient safety issue? What are the potential dangers to the patient?

Glossary

A

Abuse A misuse or improper use of something. In relationships, it is the pattern of misuse or inappropriate treatment systematically to gain control and power over another individual.

Accommodating Conflict behavior style in which an individual allows the needs of a group or team to supersede the individual's own needs. Also known as "smoothing."

Accreditation Process of officially recognizing a person or organization for meeting the standards in an area based on pre-established industry criteria.

Active euthanasia The active acceleration of death by use of drugs, for example, whether by oneself or with the aid of a physician.

Addiction Habit or behavior whose compulsive draw enslaves the individual.

Administrative law Codifies interactions between citizens and government agencies, provides certain police power to the agencies to enforce the regulations, and governs the agencies themselves.

Admissions of fact Discovery technique that asks the opposing party (in writing) to admit or deny any material fact or the authenticity of documents to be introduced into evidence at trial.

Advance directives (living wills) Means by which a patient can self-determine his or her wishes to use any artificial means to continue life if he or she is unable to communicate them in the future. These can include healthcare proxies, living wills, and durable power of attorney declarations.

Advance medical directive The treatment preferences and designation of an alternate decision maker in the event that a person should become unable to make medical decisions on his or her own behalf.

Affirmative defense A defense strategy that allows the defendant (usually provider or facility) to present the argument that the patient's condition was the result of other factors than negligence on the defendant's part.

Aggregate limit The maximum dollar amount your insurer will pay in total to settle your claims over the entire period of coverage.

Alternative dispute resolution (ADR) The procedure for settling disputes by means other than litigation.

Americans with Disabilities Act of 1990 (ADA) Laws enacted in 1990 to protect citizens with disabilities from discrimination.

Appellate court A court that hears appeals from lower court decisions; sometimes called court of appeals.

Applied ethics Application of moral principles and standards to organizations of individuals.

Arbitrator Person or persons assigned by the court to mediate in a civil suit.

Artificial insemination (AI) Injection of seminal fluid into the female vagina, which contains male sperm from a husband, partner, or other donor, to aid in conception.

Assault A threat or attempt to inflict offensive physical contact or bodily harm on a person that puts the person in immediate danger of or in apprehension of such harm or contact.

Associate practice This is a legal agreement in which physicians share staff and overhead expenses of operation but do not share in the legal responsibility or in the profits of business.

Assumption of risk A legal defense that asserts that the plaintiff was aware of risks and accepted the risks associated with the activity involved.

Avoiding Conflict behavior style in which the issue is not addressed at all or ignored.

B

Battery Bodily harm or unlawful touching of another. In the medical field, treating the patient without consent is considered battery.

Bias A preference of one thing over another, usually unfairly favoring one over another.

Bioethicists Specialists who study the ethical dilemmas resulting from advances in medical research and in science.

Bioethics Ethical dilemmas and issues that arise attributable to advances in medicine.

Brain death The irreversible loss of function of the brain, including the brain stem.

Breach of confidentiality The public revelation of confidential or privileged information without an individual's consent.

C

"Captain of the ship" doctrine An adaptation from the "borrowed servant rules," as applied to an operating room, which arose in *McConnell v. Williams,* holding the person in charge (e.g., a surgeon) responsible for all under his or her supervision, regardless of whether the "captain" is directly responsible for an alleged error or act of alleged negligence, and despite the assistants' positions as hospital employees.

CHAMPVA Acronym denoting Civilian Health and Medical Program of the Department of Veterans Affairs. Coverage designed specifically for disabled veterans and their dependents. Also known as Veterans Health Administration.

Chief complaint (CC) The main reason that the patient is being seen by a provider.

Child Abuse Prevention and Treatment Act of 1974 Law enacted in 1974 that requires the reporting of child abuse or suspected abuse.

Chromosomes Threadlike structures in the center of the cell (nucleus) that transmit the genetic information about the person.

Civil code Comprehensive collection of private laws, usually including common private laws such as those concerning contracts, torts, property, inheritance, and family issues; as opposed to corporate law.

Civil lawsuit A noncriminal lawsuit for damages, usually based in tort, contract, labor, or privacy.

Claims-made policy Insurance policy in which coverage is triggered on the date that the insured first becomes aware of the possibility of a claim and notifies the insurer. Commonly used with professional liability insurance such as medical and legal malpractice insurance.

Clearinghouse An entity that processes electronic transactions into HIPAA-standardized transactions for billing submission. May also provide billing edits for providers for claims submissions.

Clone Duplicate cell reproduced artificially from a natural, original single cell.

Code of ethics Standards of behavior, initiated by an employer or organization, defining the acceptable conduct of its members/employees (also called code of conduct).

Co-insurance This is the amount of payment that is agreed upon by the insured as his or her portion of any claims.

Collaborating Conflict behavior style in which the needs and goals of the individuals are combined to meet a common goal.

Common law Law of precedents built on a case-by-case basis and established by citing interpretation of existing laws by judges in previous suits. Also known as "judge made law."

Communicable disease Specific disease or illness that can cause an epidemic or pandemic to the general public.

Comparative negligence (or contributory negligence) A legal defense that proves the plaintiff's own actions, or lack of action, contributed to the damages done. In this defense, compensation for damages would not be prohibited but would be reduced based on the circumstance.

Compensatory damages The awarded amount given to the plaintiff in a court case to reimburse the plaintiff for loss of income or pain and suffering.

Competing Conflict behavior style in which an individual's own needs are advocated over the needs of others.

Compliance Adherence to guidelines and regulations set forth by an organization and/or a governing body.

Compliance officer The individual in an organization or practice who is designated to maintain and inspect the adherence of all areas of regulations and guidelines. (In healthcare organizations these officers perform audits and use established checks and balances to prevent fraud and abuse.)

Compliance plan Policies and procedures used to ensure that guidelines and regulations are obeyed, including auditing, monitoring, and protocol for taking action when infractions (whether deliberate or unintentional) are discovered.

Compromising Conflict behavior style in which people give and receive in a series of tradeoffs.

Confidentiality Agreement to maintain and respect the privacy of certain information disclosed. In the medical field, applies to patient privacy in particular.

Conflict The mental struggle resulting from incompatible or opposing needs, drives, wishes, or external or internal demands.

Conflict management The long-term management of disputes and conflicts, which may or may not lead to resolution.

Conflict resolution The process of ending a disagreement between two or more people in a constructive fashion for all parties involved.

Conscience clause Regulation or mandate that states that healthcare providers and/or facilities do not have to participate in procedures that are against their beliefs, such as abortions or sterilization procedures.

Consent The acknowledgment of a person (usually the patient) to the risks and alternatives involved in a treatment as well as permission for the treatment to be performed. This can be in some cases a verbal consent but in the medical field is usually a written document.

Consumer protection Laws and safeguards to protect consumers from fraudulent, unethical, or illegal practices.

Contracts An agreement voluntarily joined by two parties. These can be verbal or written and can be expressed or implied.

Control group Group of subjects in a research study who do not receive any treatment or, in some cases, are given a placebo. In testing, it is the principle of the constant that remains the same to evaluate the changes of a given experiment.

Copay A fixed amount that is determined by the health insurance policy that is paid for services to offset premiums paid by the insured.

Coroner Physician or pathologist appointed to perform autopsies and testing to determine cause of and time of death in suspicious deaths or under circumstances when no provider was in attendance of the death.

Corporation A company that is established legally and is managed by a board of directors.

Criminal law State or federal government law covering violations of written criminal code or statute.

D

Damages The actual injury or loss suffered by a defendant in a suit; usually given a monetary award by the court based on the extent of the loss or injury.

Death The permanent cessation of all biological functions that sustain a living organism.

Declarations page Portion of a liability insurance policy that provides basic information, including the name and address of the insurance agency and agent as well as contact information for the insured individual. It also states what is insured, for how much, and under which circumstances, as well as the length of time the policy is in effect.

Deductible An amount of money that is paid by the insured before the insurance company pays for services. Usually a fixed amount paid annually.

Defamation Any intentional false communication, either written or spoken, that harms a person's reputation; decreases the respect, regard, or confidence in which a person is held; or induces disparaging, hostile, or disagreeable opinions or feelings against a person.

Defendant Person or entity sued.

Defensive medicine The physician practice of ordering unnecessary tests and other procedures to protect the physician from lawsuits.

Denial Legal assertion of innocence; made only if all four elements of negligence are false.

Dereliction (of duty) A neglect or negligence of one's duty.

Direct cause In a negligence case, the correspondence between the dereliction of duty and the actual damage sustained by the plaintiff.

Disagreement A failure to agree.

Disciplinary defense insurance A type of professional liability insurance that pays legal fees for the defense of the insured during disciplinary proceedings; usually included as a feature in most professional liability policies.

Discovery Process of gathering information in preparation for trial.

Discovery rule Law or statute that states that the statute of limitations does not begin until the discovery of the diagnosis or injury.

Discrimination Treatment of a person or thing, either unsupportive or supportive, based on bias or prejudice.

Disruptive behavior Personal conduct, whether verbal or physical, that affects or that potentially may affect patient care negatively.

Do not resuscitate (DNR) Form completed by patients to indicate in advance that no means should be used to regain function of cardiopulmonary processes when these functions cease (e.g., cardiopulmonary resuscitation).

Due process Procedures or actions followed to safeguard individual rights. In the workplace, the process to safeguard an employee if he or she feels his or her rights are in jeopardy.

Durable power of attorney A type of advance medical directive in which legal documents provide the power of attorney to another person in the case of an incapacitating medical condition.

Duty In a malpractice suit, the proof of responsibility of the parties involved.

Duty-based ethics (deontology) Philosophy of ethics that focuses on performing one's duty to a group, individual, or organization.

E

Electronic health record or electronic medical record (EHR/EMR) Software systems that contain the medical records of individuals electronically under HIPAA standards for privacy and security.

Employee assistance program Program designed to help employees receive counseling for substance abuse or other issues of abuse, without fear of losing their jobs; may offer legal and financial counseling as well.

Employment-at-will The employment contract that allows an employer to fire or discharge an employee without showing just cause for the termination.

Employment Protection Acts Broad group of acts that govern handling of employees or potential employees. Generally cover the following areas: interviewing, debt collections, interest and charges, equal opportunity employment, disability act, compensation and benefit, antitrust, and antikickback.

Equal Employment Opportunity Act of 1972 Act that prohibits employment discrimination on the basis of race, color, national origin, sex, religion, age, disability, political beliefs, and marital or familial status.

Ethics Branch of philosophy that relates to morals and moral principles.

Euthanasia Termination of a life to eliminate pain and suffering related to a terminal illness, usually performed by giving a drug or agent to induce cessation of bodily functions. Also known as assisted suicide.

Excess coverage Insurance coverage that is in excess of one or more primary policies that does not pay a claim until the loss amount exceeds a specified amount. If a claim is covered by more than one policy, the second policy is said to be excess.

Exclusions A provision within an insurance policy that eliminates coverage for certain acts, types of damage, or locations.

Executive branch President of the United States or Governor of an individual state. Can propose laws, veto laws proposed by the legislature, enforce laws, and establish agencies.

F

Facilitation The process in which a third party (facilitator) assists in the resolution of a dispute.

False imprisonment A restraint of a person so as to impede his or her liberty without justification or consent.

Federal court Court having jurisdiction over cases in which the U.S. Constitution and federal statutes apply; these can be federal district courts (trial courts), district courts of appeals, or the U.S. Supreme Court.

Fee splitting An illegal act of sharing profit or compensation by a physician for referral of patients or incentives for referral of services.

Felony Serious crime punishable by relatively large fines and/or imprisonment for more than 1 year and, in some cases, death.

Fertilization Assistance in conception, most commonly performed either as artificial insemination or as in vitro fertilization to produce pregnancy.

Fraud Deliberate, intentional act to mislead for financial gain.

G

Gatekeeper A person, such as the primary care physician, or an organization that is appointed by an HMO carrier to maintain and approve services to reduce costs and unnecessary spending.

Gene therapy Process of splicing or infusing genes to replace malfunctioning genes. Alteration of the DNA of body cells to control production of a particular substance.

Good Samaritan law Law providing immunity for those who render healthcare for an emergency or disaster without reimbursement.

Group practice A medical practice with three or more physicians of the same or similar specialty, who share the same overhead and staff and practice medicine together.

H

Healthcare proxy A legal document in which an individual designates another person to make healthcare decisions if he or she is rendered incapable of making his or her wishes known.

Health Insurance Portability and Accountability Act (HIPAA) Set of laws regulated by the Office for Civil Rights (OCR) that protect and secure the information and privacy of patients. Laws that ensure a patient's rights to privacy and portability of healthcare records transmitted either nonelectronically or electronically.

Health Maintenance Organization (HMO) A type of managed care company that serves participating patients by offering services at a fixed rate within the group of participating providers and facilities. A fixed fee schedule is negotiated with the providers as well.

Hospice Organization or program involving a multidisciplinary group of medical professionals available to aid in support of the terminally ill and their families.

Human Genome Project Medical research program, sponsored by the federal government, established to map and sequence the number of genes that are within the 23 pairs of chromosomes (i.e., the 46 chromosomes) with the goal of advanced life-saving or disease-preventing treatments.

I

Implied consent Consent that is not expressly granted by a person, but rather inferred from a person's actions and the facts and circumstances of a particular situation.

***In personam* jurisdiction** A court's power to adjudicate cases filed against a specific individual, as opposed to *in rem* jurisdiction, which concerns property disputes.

***In rem* jurisdiction** A term that delineates the court's jurisdiction over property or things, including marriage, rather than over persons.

In vitro fertilization Process to assist in conception by harvesting ovum from a female and combining it with the male's sperm outside of the uterus and then implanting the fertilized embryo back into the female's uterus.

Indemnification To compensate for loss or damage; to provide financial reimbursement to an individual in case of a specified loss.

Independent contractor A person, business, or corporation that provides goods or services to another under the terms specified in a contract or within a verbal agreement, rather than as an employee.

Informed consent Same as *consent* but, in the medical field, becomes more detailed, listing and covering all possible risks and potential prognoses for having a treatment or procedure done and the alternatives available.

Inquest Investigation into a suspicious death, including autopsy and other investigations to determine time and cause of death.

Insuring agreement or clause The portion of an insurance policy in which the insurer promises to make payment to or on behalf of the insured. Insuring agreements often outline a broad scope of coverage, which is then narrowed by exclusions and definitions.

Integrity Unwavering adherence to an individual's values and principles with dedication to high standards.

Intent The willful decision to bring about a prohibited consequence.

Intentional infliction of emotional distress Type of conduct that deliberately causes severe emotional trauma to the victim.

Intentional tort A category of torts that describes a civil wrong resulting from an intentional act on the part of another person or entity.

Interrogatory Pretrial set of written questions that must be answered in writing under oath and returned within a given time frame.

Invasion of privacy The wrongful intrusion into private affairs with which the perpetrator or the public has no concern.

Involuntary euthanasia The active effort to end the life of a patient who has not explicitly requested aid in dying. This term is most often used with respect to patients who are in a persistent vegetative state and who probably will never recover consciousness.

J

Judicial branch Federal constitutional court system; one of the three parts of the U.S. Federal Government; interprets legislation and determines its constitutionality, applying it to specific cases. May overrule cases presented on appeal from lower courts.

Jurisdiction Authority given by law to a court to try cases and rule on legal matters within a particular geographic area and/or over certain types of legal cases.

Justice-based ethics Ethical philosophy based on all individuals having equal rights.

L

Law The foundation of statutes, rules, and regulations that govern people, relationships, behaviors, and interactions with the state, society, and federal government.

Legislative branch The U.S. House of Representatives and Senate and any similar state legislature that develops statutory law.

Liability Obligations under law arising from civil actions or torts.

Liable Legal responsibility for a person's own actions.

Libel Written, printed, or other visual communication that harms another person's reputation.

Limited Liability Company (LLC) A legally structured company in which the members of the corporation cannot be held personally liable for the debts or actions of the company or another party in the company.

Litigious Highly inclined to sue.

Living will A document in which the patient states his or her wishes regarding medical treatment, especially treatment that sustains or prolongs life by extraordinary means, in the event that the patient becomes mentally incompetent or unable to communicate.

M

Malfeasance The performance of an illegal act.

Malpractice The failure of a professional to meet the standard of conduct that a reasonable and prudent member of the profession would exercise in similar circumstances; it results in harm.

Mediation The process by which a neutral third party who is trained in mediation techniques facilitates and assists in resolving a dispute.

Medicaid Federal program administered by each individual state that provides healthcare coverage for the indigent and/or medically needy patients.

Medical ethics Principles based on the medical profession that determine moral behavior.

Medical law Laws that are prescribed specifically pertaining to the medical field.

Medical practice acts Laws defined by each of the states that regulate the licensing and medical laws for that state and define the scope of practice for licensed and unlicensed individuals in the healthcare field.

Medicare Federal program that provides medical insurance coverage to members older than age 65 or to those who are deemed permanently disabled.

Medicare fraud Providing false information to claim medical reimbursements beyond the scope of payment for actual healthcare services rendered.

Misdemeanor Lesser crime punishable by usually modest fines or penalties established by the state or federal government and/or imprisonment of less than 1 year.

Misfeasance Poor performance of a duty or action, causing damage.

Morals Standards of right and wrong. Moral values that govern behavior and thinking based on principles of what is right and wrong. The norms of measuring right from wrong.

N

National Organ Transplant Act (NOTA) Act of Congress that established the Organ Procurement and Transplantation Network (OPTN) to maintain a national registry for organ matching and to provide grants to qualified organ procurement organizations.

Negative conflict Conflict that has devolved into disruptive behaviors or violence.

Negligence The failure to use such care as a reasonably prudent and careful person would use under similar circumstances; an act of omission or failure to do what a person of ordinary prudence would have done under similar circumstances.

Negotiation Any communication used in an attempt to achieve a goal, approval, or action by another.

Nominal damages A small payment or award given by the court.

Nonfeasance A failure to perform an action when needed.

Nontherapeutic research Medical research in which the test subjects are not necessarily suffering from a disease or the particular disease that the study is researching, and therefore the subjects are not receiving a direct medical benefit from participating in the study.

O

Occupational Safety and Health Act of 1970 Act that defines and enforces safety regulations for the health and protection of employees in the workplace.

Occupational Safety and Health Administration (OSHA) Federal agency within the Department of Labor that designs, regulates, and monitors standards for employee safety.

Occurrence basis policy An insurance policy that covers claims taking place during the policy period, regardless of when claims are made.

Office for Civil Rights (OCR) Federal office established to uphold the rights of individuals, regarding rights to privacy and standards of care. Enforces the HIPAA regulations.

Office of Inspector General (OIG) Independent agency that functions under the Department of Justice to investigate and protect the integrity of the Department of Health and Human Services (HHS) and their recipients, as well as welfare programs.

P

Palliative care Literally meaning to ease or comfort; the care provided to terminally ill patients to alleviate symptoms and discomfort suffered while dying.

Passive euthanasia The act of allowing a patient to die without medical intervention.

Patient Self-Determination Act Federal law that requires all healthcare institutions receiving Medicare or Medicaid funds to provide patients with written information about their right under state law to execute advance directives. The written information must clearly state the institution's policies on withholding or withdrawing life-sustaining treatment.

Persistent vegetative state (PVS) Condition characterized by the irreversible cessation of the higher brain functions. Usually as a result of damage to the cerebral cortex.

Placebo Nontherapeutic drug or agent given to a control group. (Commonly referred to as a "sugar pill.")

Plaintiff The person or entity bringing a suit or claim.

Policy jacket Binder or folder containing an insurance policy; in many instances it lists provisions common to several types of policies.

Positive conflict The idea that healthy discussion can happen in the face of a disagreement, regardless of differing personalities, education levels, or responsibilities.

Postmortem Examination that is performed on an individual after death.

Premium The amount of money an insurer charges to provide the coverage described in the policy.

Primary care physician (PCP) A designated provider that oversees the care and manages the healthcare services for an individual.

Prior acts coverage Insurance coverage for incidents that occur before the start of the policy but whose claims are made during the policy period.

Professional corporation (PC) A specific legal company structure that is designed for individuals providing professional services to their clients, such as lawyers, physicians, or architects.

Protected health information (PHI) Information about any individual that is identifiable and private about that individual (e.g., Social Security number, date of birth). Public information (such as name and address) is not considered PHI.

Public duties Responsibility of healthcare providers to report vital information to the necessary agencies as necessary for the welfare of the general public.

Punitive damages An award granted by the courts to punish the defendant for the damages done based on a malicious or intentional act.

Q

Quasi-intentional tort A voluntary act that directly causes damage to a person's privacy or emotional well-being, but without the intent to injure or to cause distress.

***Qui tam* (whistleblower)** In Latin meaning "who as well"; this is the term used for a private citizen who exposes and sues a company or organization that is violating a law and/or breaching a contract with the government. In such cases, the whistleblower may be entitled to a percentage amount or settlement reward for the uncovering of the illegal action.

R

Release of tortfeasor Law that asserts that once the person causing damage (the tortfeasor) is released from further liability in a previous suit's settlement, he or she cannot be held liable in a subsequent suit.

Request for production of documents A discovery tool whereby requests are submitted to the opposing party to produce specific documents or items that are pertinent to the issues of the case.

Res ipsa loquitur In Latin: "the thing speaks for itself." Legal indication that there is clear proof that the defendant had the responsibility (duty) to the patient and that the injury would not and could not have occurred without the negligence of the defendant.

Res judicata Law that forbids suing a subsequent time for the same damages once a case has already been resolved.

Respondeat superior Legal doctrine stating that, in many circumstances, an employer is responsible for the actions of employees performed within the course of their employment.

Rights-based ethics Philosophy of ethics based on theory of the rights of each individual (autonomy).

S

Sanctions Penalties that can be levied on an individual for violating a policy or rule. (Can also mean permission or agreement in other contexts.)

Scope of practice Officially sanctioned description of the specific procedures, actions, and processes that are permitted for a licensed or nonlicensed professional; based on the specific state's laws for education and experience requirements, plus demonstrated competency. Established by the state's laws, licensing board, and/or agency regulations.

Self-insurance A system in which a business sets aside an amount of money to provide for any losses that occur—losses that would ordinarily be covered under an insurance program. The monies that would typically be used for premium payments are added to this special fund for payment of losses incurred.

Settlement Legal agreement that is reached between two parties in a civil matter.

Sexual assault Any type of sexual activity to which a person does not agree.

Sexual harassment Use of power or intimidation over an individual for sexual favors; unwanted or unwelcomed sexual advances and actions or behaviors with sexual implications or innuendoes leading another individual to feel uncomfortable or offended.

Slander Spoken or verbal communication in which one person discusses another in terms that harm that person's reputation.

SOAP Acronym for documentation, standing for Subjective, Objective, Assessment, and Plan.

Sole proprietorship A single professional-owned business in which an individual employs other professionals in the same field. In medical practice, single physician-owned practice that employs other physicians to work for the practice.

Solo practice Single owner/operator of the company or business. In the medical field, this would represent a single physician practice.

Specialist In the medical field, an individual who has undergone further specific training in a certain discipline and practices medicine in that discipline, such as dermatology or endocrinology.

Standard of care The average knowledge and expertise that one can expect from a healthcare professional in the same area or field and with the same base of training.

Standards of practice Basic skill and care expected of healthcare professionals in the same or similar branch of medicine; based on what another medical professional would deem to be "appropriate" in similar circumstances (also known as standards of care).

Stare decisis In Latin: "to stand by the things decided" or to adhere to a decided case; condition in which, once a court rules, that decision becomes law for other cases. Also known as *precedent*.

Stark laws Laws designed to maintain the integrity of the medical field; include antitrust and antikickback laws to prevent physicians from gaining financially from solicitation of services or monopolization of services.

State Supreme Court Highest court in any given state in the U.S. court system.

Statute of limitations Defense against a tort action; requires that a claim be filed within a specific amount of time of discovering that a wrong has been committed.

Stem cells Cells of the body that can control the production of specialized cells by becoming other types of cells as needed during growth or healing.

Sterilization Any procedure performed to permanently prevent reproduction.

Subpoena A court order for records or appearance in court for a trial case.

Subpoena *duces tecum* A Latin phrase meaning "under penalty take it with you." Used in medicolegal matters to subpoena a provider or facility to bring the defendant's file or records with them when appearing in court.

T

Tail coverage A provision of a claims-made liability policy that allows the insured to purchase coverage for claims made during a specified time period after the end of the policy.
It covers the claim as long as the incident occurred during the time the policy was in place.

Terminally ill Illness with an expected survival of less than 6 months.

Thanatology The study of the effects of death and dying, especially the investigation of ways to lessen the suffering and address the needs of the terminally ill and their survivors.

The Joint Commission The organization that accredits hospitals and other healthcare organizations.

Therapeutic research Medical research performed on chronically or terminally ill patients who may benefit from the agent being tested.

Third party payer Usually refers to the insurance company but can be any other person or organization that is responsible for the medical care coverage of a patient.

Tolerance Respect for others whose beliefs, practices, race, religions, or customs may differ from one's own.

Tort A wrongful act, not including a breach of contract or trust, that results in injury to another's person, property, reputation, or the like, and for which the injured party is entitled to compensation.

Trespass An unlawful intrusion that interferes with one's person, property (called "chattels"), or land.

TRICARE Government medical program for active duty military and their dependents as well as coverage for military retirees (after 20 or more years of service).

U

Umbrella coverage Liability insurance policy that provides protection against claims that are not covered, or are in excess of the amount covered, under a basic liability insurance policy.

Uniform Anatomical Gift Act Legislation that allows a person to make an anatomical gift at the time of death by the use of a signed document such as a will or driver's license—the person can donate all or part of his or her body for medical education, scientific research, or organ transplantation.

Uniform Determination of Death Act (UDDA) Model state legislation that has since been adopted by most U.S. states and is intended "to provide a comprehensive and medically sound basis for determining death in all situations."

Uniform Rights of the Terminally Ill Act Legislation that allows a person to declare a living will specifying that, if the situation arises, he or she does not wish to be kept alive through life support if terminally ill or in a coma. The patient may also obtain a healthcare power of attorney. This power of attorney appoints an agent to make medical decisions for the patient in case the patient becomes incompetent.

Unintentional tort An unintended wrong against another person.

United States Supreme Court Highest court in the United States, having ultimate judicial authority within the United States to interpret and decide questions of federal law. It is head of the judicial branch of the United States Government.

Utilitarianism Ethical theory based on the greatest good for the greatest number (also known as cost/benefit analysis).

V

Values Principles that individuals choose to follow in their lives.

Vicarious liability The liability of an employer for the actions of its designated agents. Vicarious liability can result from the acts of independent agents, partners, independent contractors, and employees.

Virtue-based ethics Ethical theory or philosophy that relies on the principle that individuals share and will hold as their governing principle values of moral behavior and character.

Vital statistics (public) Community-wide recording of individual key human events such as births, deaths, marriages, and divorces.

Voluntary euthanasia Conscious medical act that results in the death of a patient who has given consent.

W

Writ of certiorari Order a higher court issues to review the decision and proceedings in a lower court and determine whether there were any irregularities.

Wrongful discharge A situation when an employee alleges cause that the employment contract or agreement was terminated unjustly or unfairly and therefore the employment contract was breached. The termination of an employee without just cause, without following proper procedures or without due process.

Index

Page numbers followed by "f" indicate figures, "t" indicate tables, and "b" indicate boxes.